W9-AIT-241

Contents

Acknowledgments

Sincere appreciation is extended to all the wonderful folks at Schiffer Publishing who graciously helped me behind the scenes, thus making this book a reality in a short period of time.

I could never write a book without thanking my husband, Terry; not only for his patience, but for hauling my clothing to its destination to be photographed, helping me sort it once we arrived, quickly changing mannequins, and driving home two hours in a snow storm.

To my mother, Marie, my son, Clint, and my daughter, Amber, thank you for taking care of my two "little ones," Sabrina and Lexie, while I was away changing mannequins.

And last, but certainly not least, to Peter and Nancy Schiffer; you're great, as always. Thank You.

Introduction

No single volume can depict all the styles of a particular era, whether it be furniture, glassware, pottery or jewelry— and fashions are definitely no exception. Three years ago, when I wrote *'50s Popular Fashions*, I stated that it was impossible to capture of essence of the entire decade in one volume. Now that the second volume is complete, I have to say the same thing. Two volumes are still not enough! Unless, by some luck, I stumble upon an attic filled with designer clothing from the 1950s, I don't plan on working on the third volume any time soon. But one never knows. It can happen!

Over the last few years, vintage clothing has really become a hot property! Collectors and dealers have become very specialized. Categories like vintage denim, Hawaiian shirts, bowling shirts and men's gabardine top the list. Other categories, especially hand-painted neckties and Western wear is also extremely desirable. Tailored suits, Dior-inspired dresses, sexy Italian-styled capri pants and tight-fitting sweaters are sought after by vintage clothing enthusiasts.

Because of the current demand for vintage clothing, prices are escalating. Items from the 1950s are not as easy to find as they were five years ago, as the law of supply and demand comes into effect. But an occasional sleeper is still out there waiting to be found, That, my friends, is what makes this "passion" so exciting.

Wearing vintage has become very trendy. Major cities across the country have shows solely devoted to vintage clothing. Major auction houses have vintage clothing sales a few times a year. Fashion designers shop the vintage clothing shows searching for ideas for their upcoming lines. Certain actors, actresses and rock stars wear vintage clothing. No longer is there a stigma attached to wearing "old clothes." Vintage is the "in" thing and here to stay! So it's *Fifties Forever!*

Fifties Forever!

Popular Fashions for Men, Women, Boys & Girls

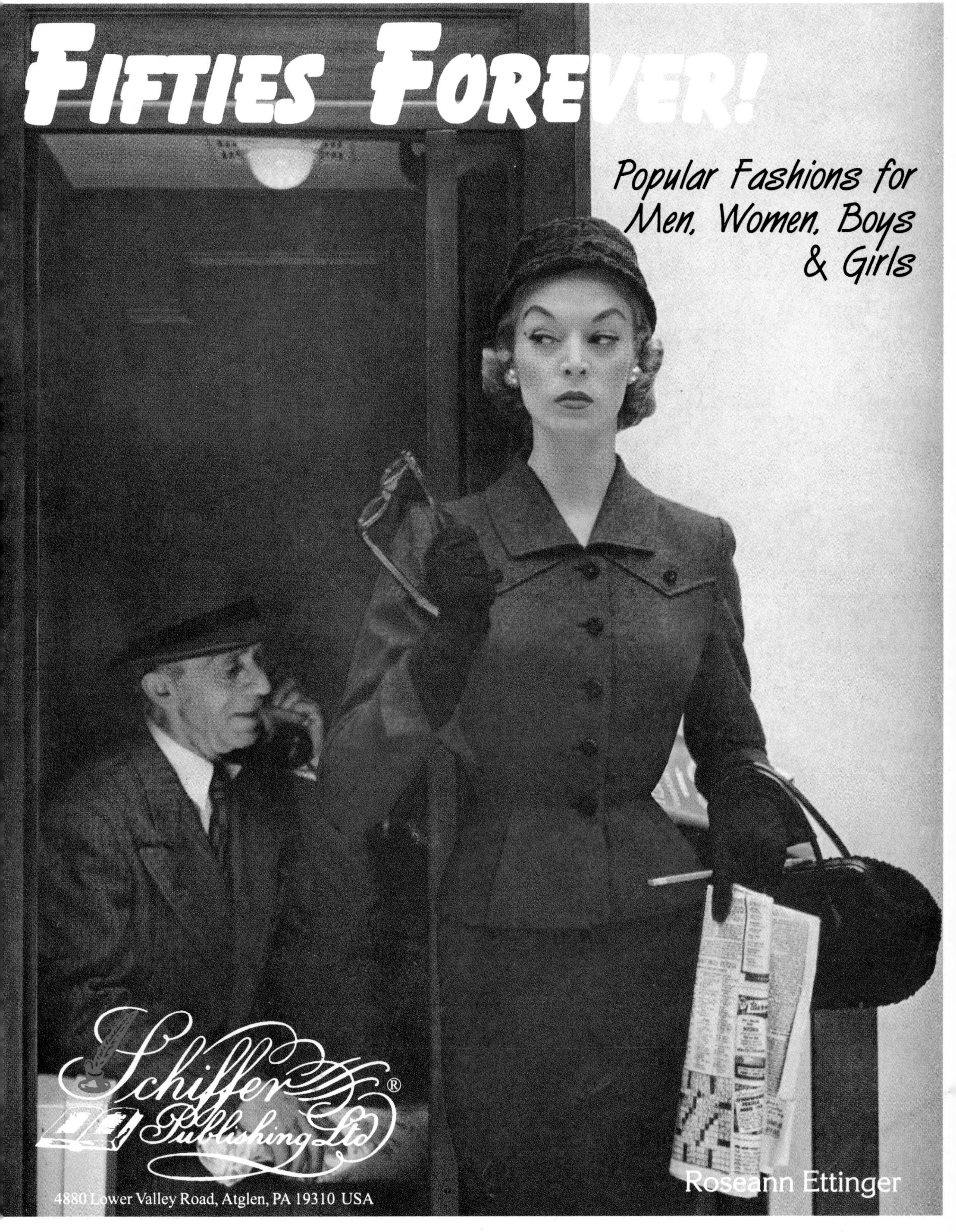

Roseann Ettinger

Schiffer® Publishing Ltd
4880 Lower Valley Road, Atglen, PA 19310 USA

Dedication

To all my friends, fans and customers who made *'50s Popular Fashions* a hit and encouraged me to work on a second volume.

Designed by Bonnie M. Hensley
Typeset in VanDijk/Korinna

ISBN: 0-7643-0640-5
Printed in China
1 2 3 4

Published by Schiffer Publishing Ltd.
4880 Lower Valley Road Atglen, PA 19310
Phone: (610) 593-1777; Fax: (610) 593-2002
E-mail: Schifferbk@aol.com

In Europe, Schiffer books are distributed by
Bushwood Books
6 Marksbury Avenue Kew Gardens
Surrey TW9 4JF England
Phone: 44(0)181-392-8585
Fax: 44(0) 181-392-9876
E-mail: Bushwd@aol.com

Please write for a free catalog. This book may be purchased from the publisher. Please include $3.95 for shipping. Please try your bookstore first. We are interested in hearing from authors with book ideas on related subjects.

Chapter 1

Fashions For Women

Dresses

Tucks, gathers and peplums embellished the dresses of the early 1950s, but as the decade progressed rapid changes occurred and a kaleidscope of styles filtered there way into the fashion world. The shirtwaist dress, either designed for day or evening wear, was extremely stylish. For daytime, cotton, jersey and Nylon were popular fabric choices. For evening wear, Rayon, taffeta, silk and assorted blends fit the bill. If the dress fabric was a solid color, it would have texture or good draping qualities. Lace, elaborate beadwork or rhinestones were added for extra excitement. Printed fabric was extremely exciting in the 1950s. Anything from polka dots to floral prints as well as abstract and novelty prints were offered. Designer fabrics entered the fashion scene in this decade, and artist inspired prints were extremely chic.

Sheath dresses in tweedy mixtures of acetate and Nylon were stylish in the mid-1950s. Coat dresses, long-torso dresses, jumpers and mix & match separates were also made of this type of fabric. In the Fall of 1954, the polo-shirt dress made of jersey knit became a hit.

Unusual collar treatment was found throughout the decade, not only on dresses, but suits, coats, blouses and sweaters as well. Peter Pan, wing, mandarin, middy, man-tailored, detachable, pilgrim and shawl collars were a few of the most popular. For more fashion excitement, extra attention was also paid to pockets and unusual pocket treatment was common on dresses, suits and coats. Jumbo patch pockets were stylish in addition to double flap pockets. The proportionately enlarged pockets were sometimes trimmed with braid work or piping. Flap pockets were sometimes beaded or buttons added for extra ornamentation. Collars, cuffs and pockets were also outlined in contrasting colors or completely different fabrics. For example, a three-piece wool tweed suit could be outlined in a solid gabardine. Another example could be a Nylon lace dress trimmed with acetate.

Ensembles were another 1950s favorite. Jacket dresses, consisting of a dress and matching bolero jacket or fitted blazer were common as well as dresses and companion coats. The coats would either be full-length or three-quarter length. The coat fabric differed from the dress fabric but occasionally the coat was lined with the identical fabric as the dress.

By the late 1950s, the Empire sheath dress was in vogue and designed in many different ways. The che-mise dress, the tunic dress, the sack dress and the trapeze dress were all favorites of the stylish woman of the late 1950s and advertised heavily in leading fashion magazines.

With a few exceptions, the birth of new designs and continual changes in women's fashion can be created to master designer Christian Dior. A "Paris Extra" from RCA Communications featured in *Mademoiselle* in September of 1954 had this to say about designers and up-coming fashion trends:

Dior gave us curves in his New Look in 1947. He now dispenses with them in his "H" line 1955. Though he cannot change nature, illusion is complete: small head, long slender torso ending at hips (hips are focus of everything with skirt straight or pleated or flared). Bosoms are bound up instead of down, as in Twenties—more like eighteenth century Fragonard paintings. His new patented bras raise bosom two inches. He de-emphasizes collars on coats, replacing with draped folds. His newest suit has riding-habit jacket, knuckle length, standing away from slim skirt. His blouses all over-blouses...spread of Chanel influence seen in tube dresses, tank decolletages, cardigans, jerseys, middies, illusion of lower waist...coats every type, full-length predominating, bulky greatcoats, flared princess coats, slim reefers to slender, tapered coats, also satin or lamé trench coats are here. Pale coats over black dresses...many suits with short fitted jackets barely reaching hipbone, also windbreak jackets. Couture fur-mad with fur-lined fur coats, fur-lined cloth coats, fur accessories, fur trimming...Long slim torso universal dress silhouette. Long skinny sleeves add to slim look. Many dresses unbelted, others have wide belts giving illusion of lower waist...After-five dresses mostly full-skirted below long, molded torso...Fath revives Chanel tank-top chemise dress...Short or long evening dresses but anklebone length. Balenciaga and Dior show short in front, longer back. New, naive decolletage: high, straight across, strapped...coat suit fabrics: much tweed, also fleece, zibeline, duvetyn, chinchilla, broadcloth, flannel...After-five dresses: velveteen, velvet, lamé jersey, black crepe. For evening: satin supreme, much lace, some chiffon...colors: black overwhelming for day, then fur browns, lighter grays to black oxford, red range important, gamut of blues, some amethyst and grape, evening entire pink rose to red range, also icy pastels. Newest—sharp yellow satin...Hats mainly small, worn straight, some entirely covering hair or hugging back of head. Sailors all sizes...Long ropes of pearls and other beads. Elaborate Far Eastern jeweled bib necklaces, chandelier earrings, Fath's huge rhinestone buckles and his enormous cuff links sure to invade America.—B.T.B.

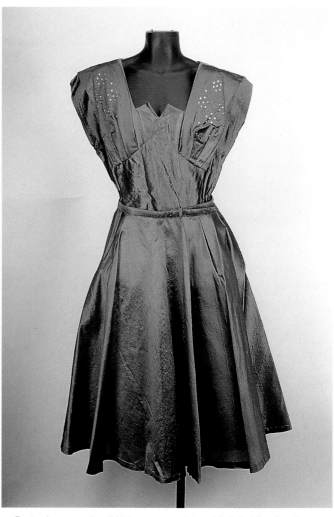

Party dress made of iridescent acetate with full skirt, fitted bodice and cap sleeves, decorated with rhinestones, no label. $35-50

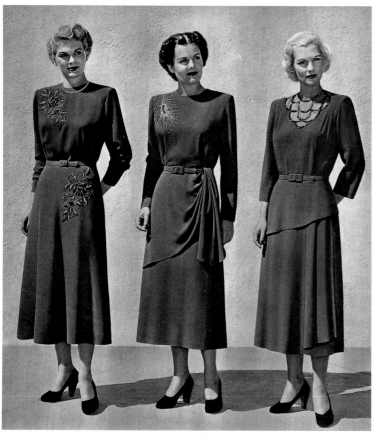

The 1940s look was carried over into the early 1950s. These exquisite rayon crepe dresses, accented with embroidery and bugle beads, were offered for sale in 1950.

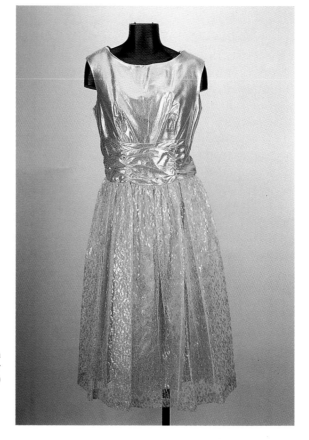

Sleeveless gold party dress of imitation gold lamé top with acetate lace over taffeta, no label. $35-50

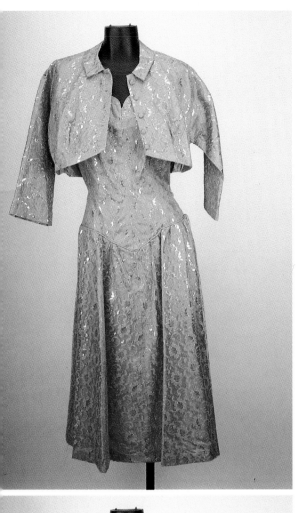

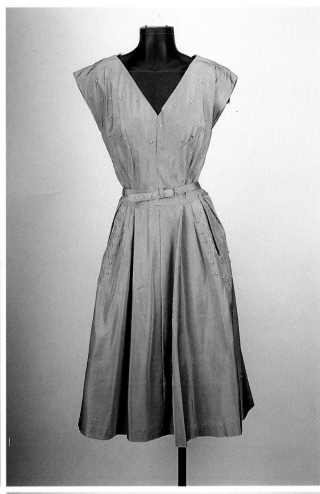

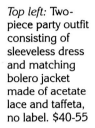

Top left: Two-piece party outfit consisting of sleeveless dress and matching bolero jacket made of acetate lace and taffeta, no label. $40-55

Top right: V-neck party dress with belted waist and cap sleeves, accented with rhinestones and pearls, made of iridescent acetate, no label. $35-45

Bottom left: Nylon party dress of white chiffon, printed with large yellow roses. Matching bolero jacket made of rayon. Labeled An Original Jr. Theme New York. $40-50

Bottom right: White nylon chiffon party dress with v-neck, accented with flocked rose decoration and large, red acetate waistband, no label. $35-45

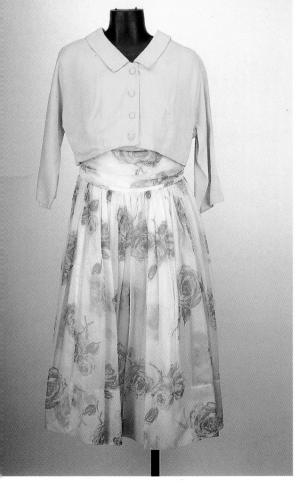

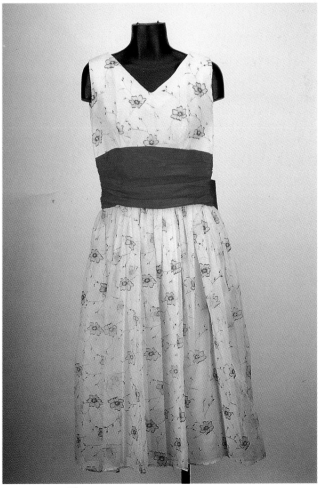

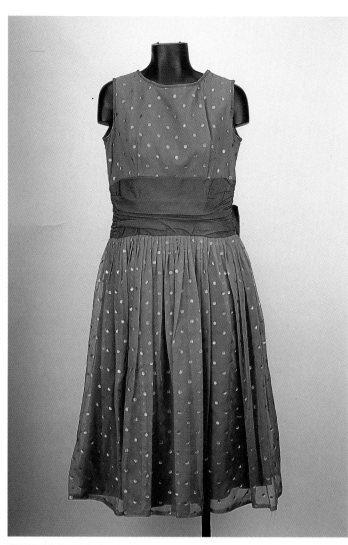

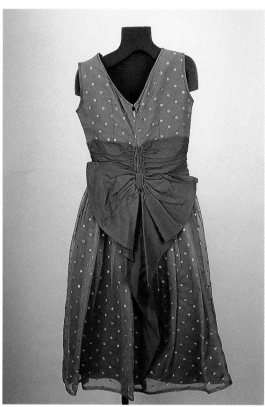

Green nylon chiffon party dress, lined in acetate, with hand-printed gold polka dots and large green acetate waistband. Back view shows large decorative bow, no label. $35-45

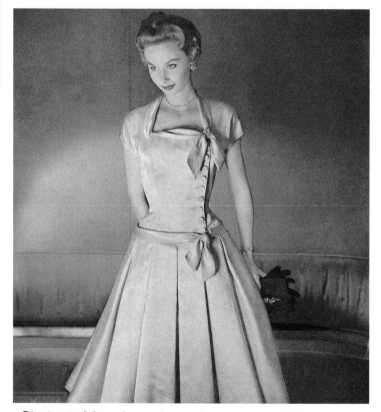

Dior-inspired dress designed with a long-torso by R & K Originals advertised for sale in December of 1954.

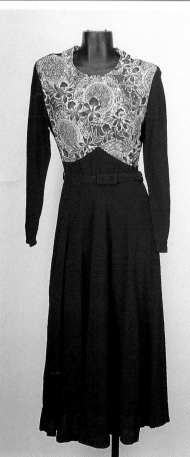

Navy blue rayon crepe dress with floral printed bodice, no label. $40-50

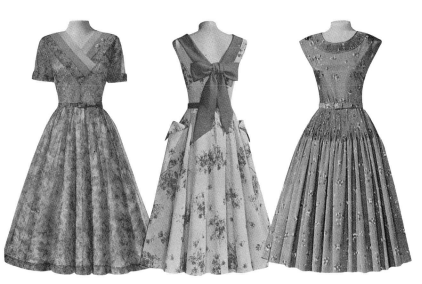

Printed rayon dresses designed for the Spring of 1955.

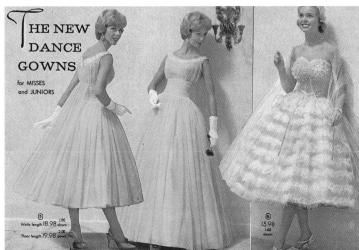

Nylon party dresses in waltz length and floor length popular in 1959.

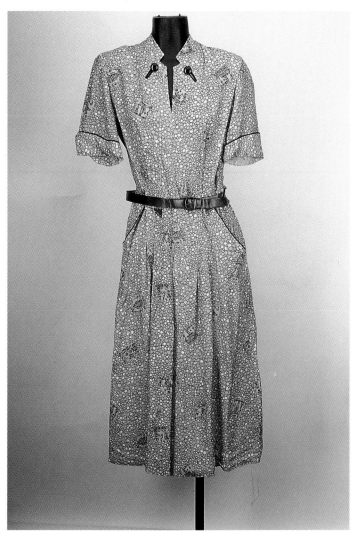

Mauve colored rayon dress with pebbled design and piped trim, navy vinyl belt, labeled Cáy Artley. $35-45

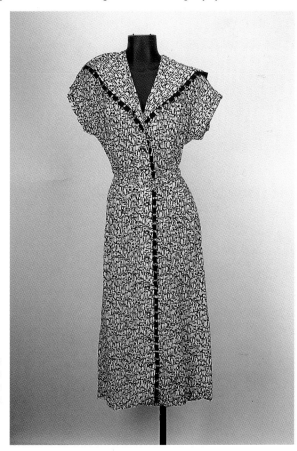

Black and white sheer rayon crepe dress printed with ladies and umbrellas accented with black trim and rhinestone buttons, no label. $30-40

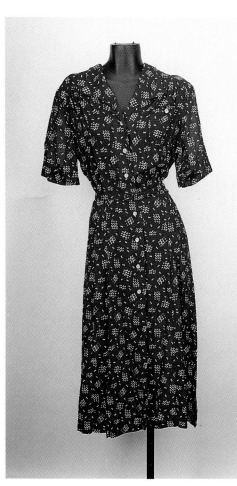

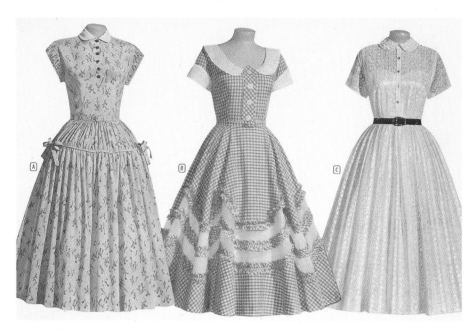

Ladies' dresses designed with the "Little Girl" look, a popular trend in the mid-1950s.

Navy blue and white shirtwaist dress made of
Bemberg rayon yarn, geometric print, labeled
The House of Shroyers. $30-40

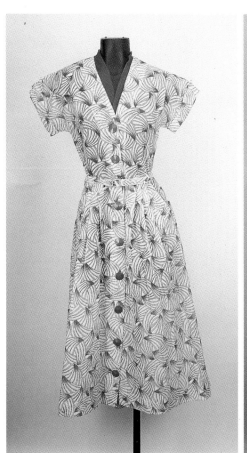

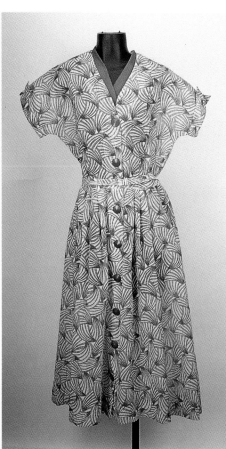

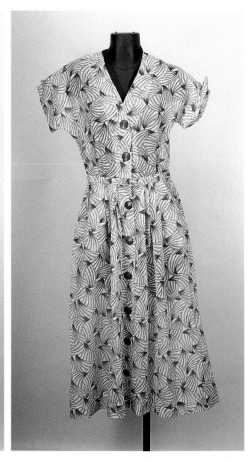

Shirtwaist dresses made of textured nylon with abstract prints, labeled The House of Shroyers. $25-35 each

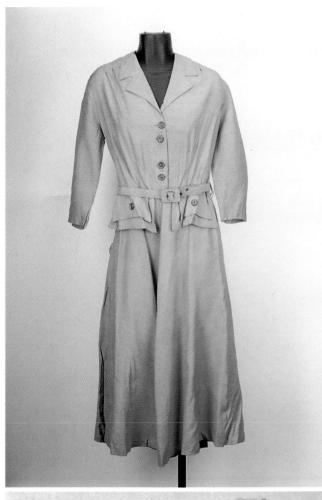
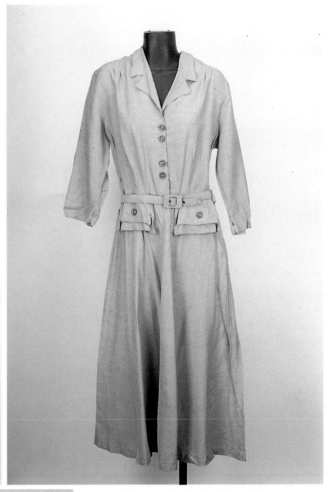

Classic tailoring is defined in these two rayon dresses, labeled Quaker Lady Frock. $45-55 each

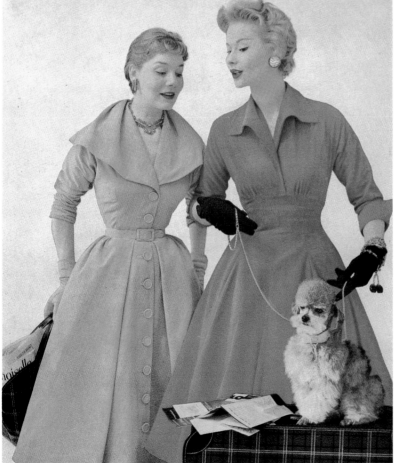

Two dresses made of fine-ribbed corduroy designed by Frances Prisco for Ted Brown, New York, in 1954. Notice the unusual collar treatment on both dresses.

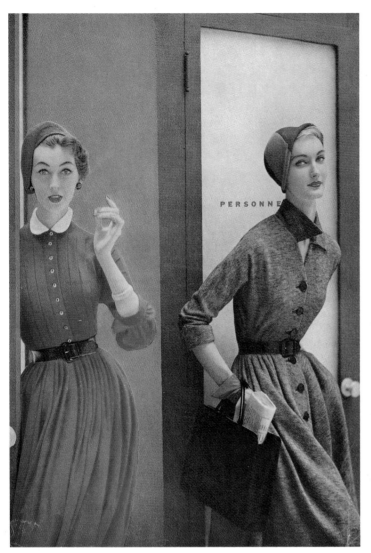

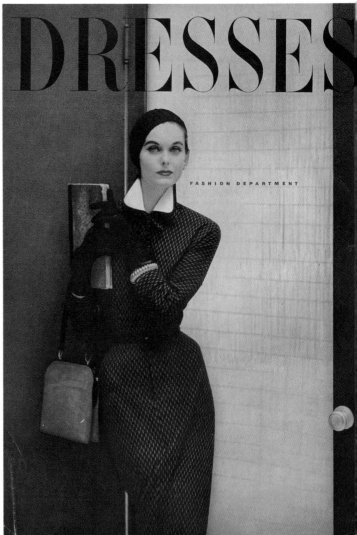

Two classic belted shirtwaist dresses - a fashion must for Milady's wardrobe throughout the 1950s. These two examples were featured in *Charm* magazine in 1954.

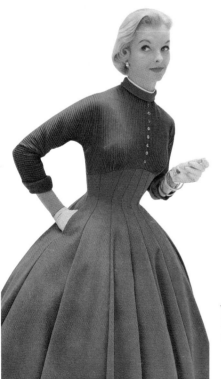

Top right: Belted sheath dress with stand-up collar - a fashionable look for the Fall of 1954 advertised in *Charm* magazine.

Bottom right: Off-white gabardine shirtwaist dress with small print, black vinyl belt, styled by Lenny. $30-40

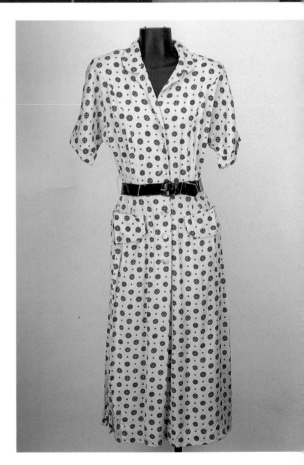

Wool flannel dress by Jonathan Logan advertised in *Charm* magazine in the Fall of 1954.

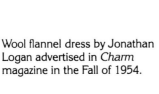

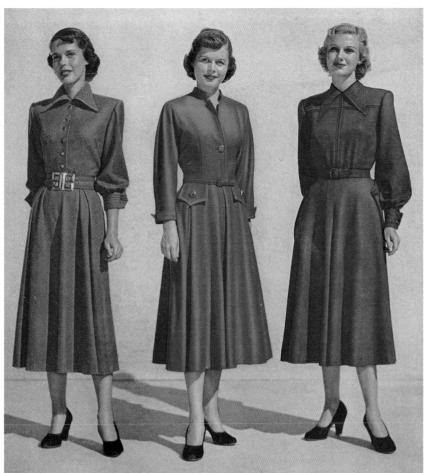

Classic shirtwaist dresses from 1950 designed with wing collars and standing notched collar available in wool crepe, non-crush rayon or rayon gabardine.

Red gabardine shirtwaist dress with small print, black vinyl belt, styled by Lenny. $30-40

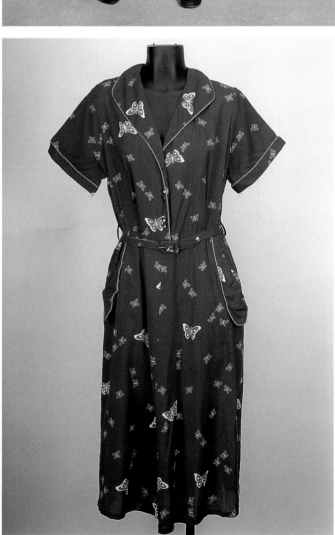

Brown dress made of butcher rayon with butterfly print, orange piping, styled by Marilyn of Philadelphia. $25-35

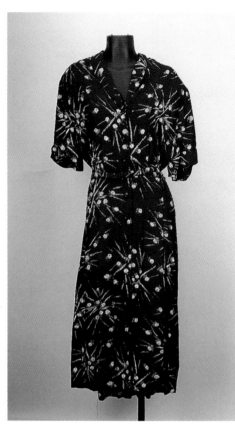

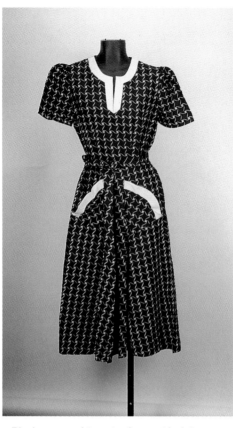

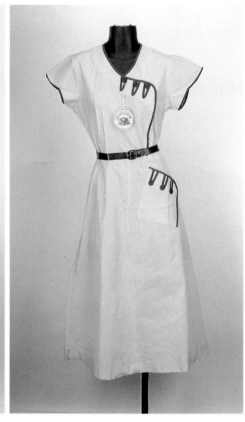

Navy blue rayon day dress with small floral print, belted waist, labeled The House of Shroyers. $35-45

Black cotton shirtwaist dress with daisy print, designed with textured cotton collar and pocket trim, labeled Sue Sherry, Division of Sherman Manufacturing Company. $25-35

Short sleeve, waffled cotton shirtwaist dress, accented with harmonizing trim and button decoration, labeled Fruit of the Loom. $30-40

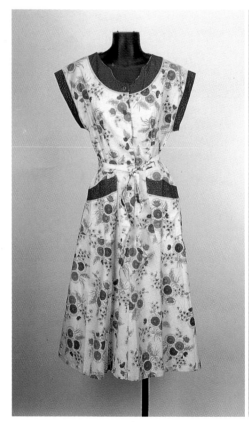

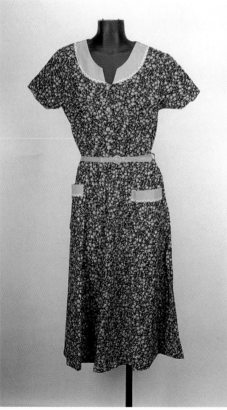

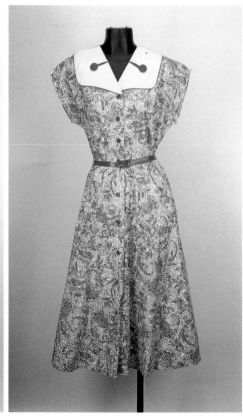

Short sleeve cotton shirtwaist dress with abstract floral pattern, accented with purple textured cotton, labeled Fruit of the Loom. $25-35

Black cotton shirtwaist dress with small pink floral print and solid color textured trim, labeled Fruit of the Loom. $25-35

Gray and white cotton dress with abstract floral print, accented with white textured cotton collar and red piping, labeled Simplicity Frock. $25-35

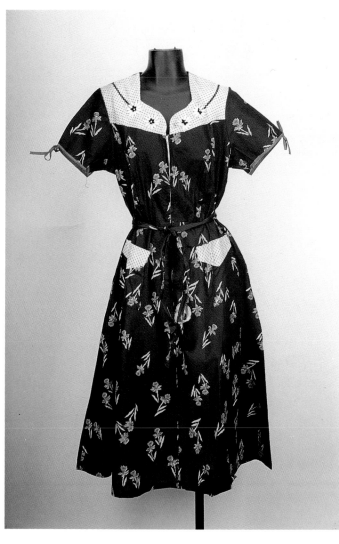

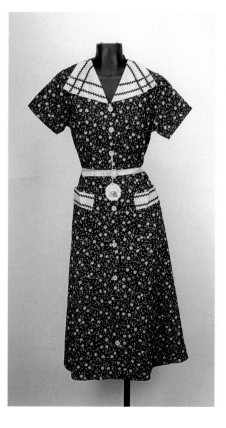

Black cotton house dress with small pink floral print and pink textured cotton collar and pockets, accented with black rick-rack, labeled Fruit of the Loom. $25-35

Black cotton day dress with floral print and organdy dotted Swiss trim accented with floral appliques, labeled Fruit of the Loom. $25-35

Plaid, satin stripe and gingham dresses offered for sale from Montgomery Ward in 1953.

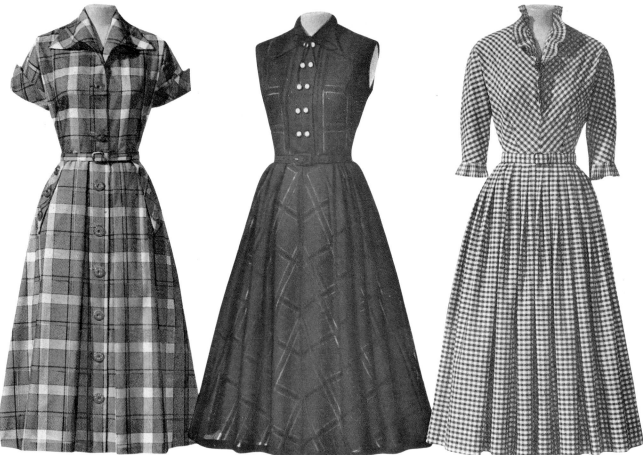

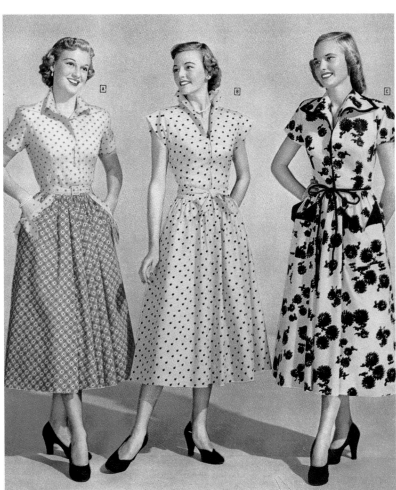

Cotton broadcloth dresses in cheerful colors designed with wing, Queen Ann and pointed roll collars offered for sale in 1950.

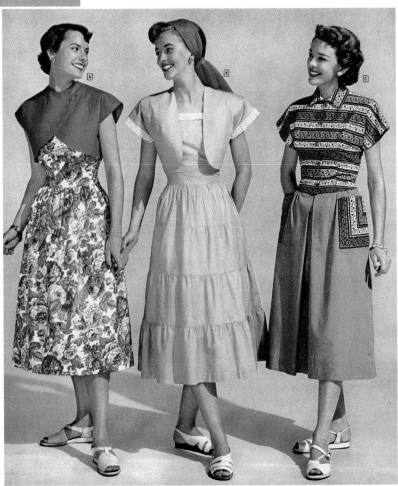

Sunback dresses styled with either bolero or fitted jackets made of solid color or printed cottons fashionable in the Summer of 1950.

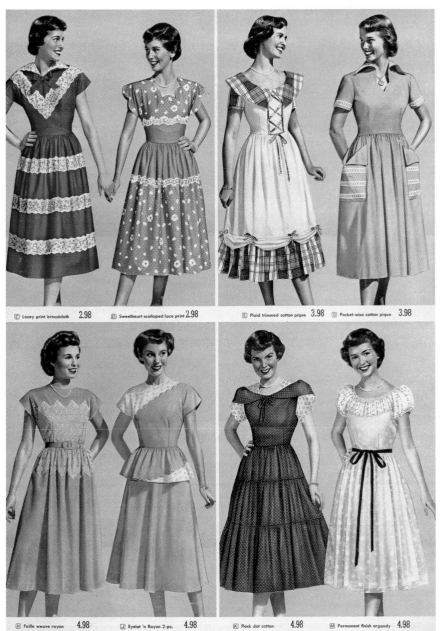

| C Lacey print broadcloth 2.98 | D Sweetheart scalloped lace print 2.98 | E Plaid trimmed cotton pique 3.98 | G Pocket-wise cotton pique 3.98 |

| H Faille weave rayon 4.98 | J Eyelet 'n Rayon 2-pc. 4.98 | K Flock dot cotton 4.98 | M Permanent finish organdy 4.98 |

Stylish ladies' day dresses from 1950 made of cotton broadcloth, cotton pique, rayon faille and organdy.

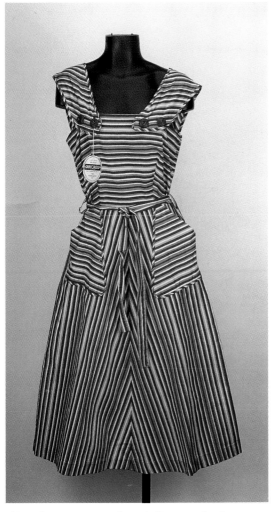

Sleeveless cotton sundress in five-toned stripes, labeled Fruit of the Loom. $20-30

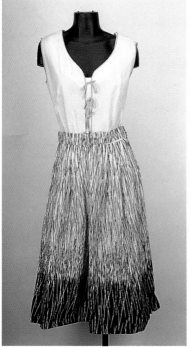

Sleeveless cotton day dress with white textured cotton top and tri-colored abstract printed bottom, styled by Marilyn of Philadelphia. $20-30

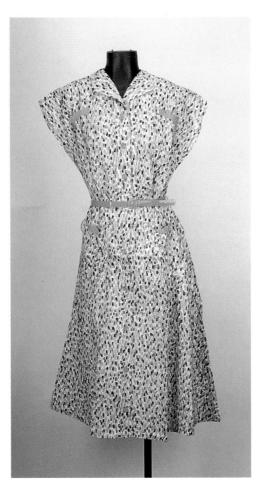

Two identical cotton dresses in four-toned color combinations with solid color pocket ornamentation and plastic belts, labeled Fruit of the Loom. $20-30 each

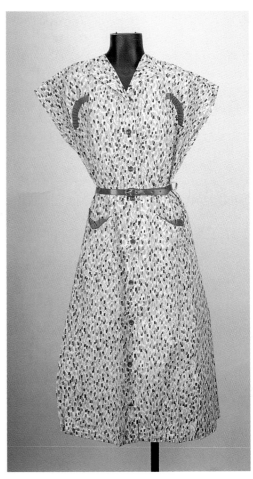

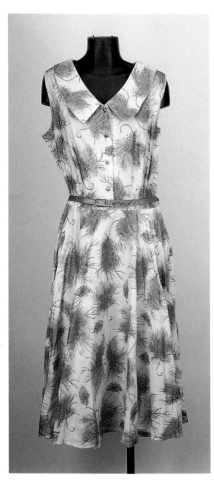

Sleeveless cotton shirtwaist dress with printed gold twig design, trimmed in gold piping, accented with a gold vinyl belt, labeled Fruit of the Loom. $20-30

Two-piece cotton outfit consisting of sleeveless top and circle skirt with solid color and paisley print design, no label. $25-35

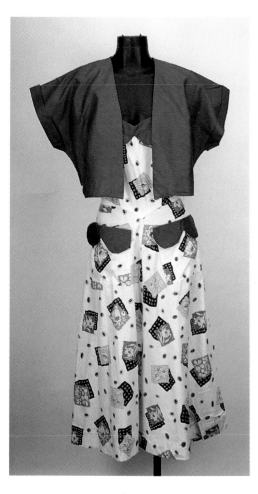

Sleeveless cotton sundress with matching bolero jacket, in a floral print with solid color trim, labeled Sue Sherry. $30-40

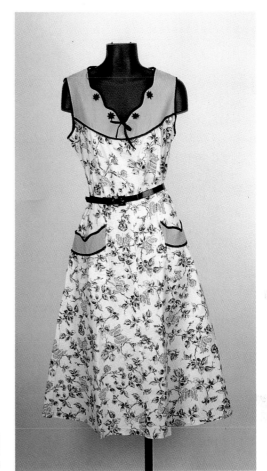

Two sleeveless, cotton shirtwaist dresses with floral prints and solid color yokes and pockets, accented with black piping and floral appliques, labeled Fruit of the Loom. $25-35 each

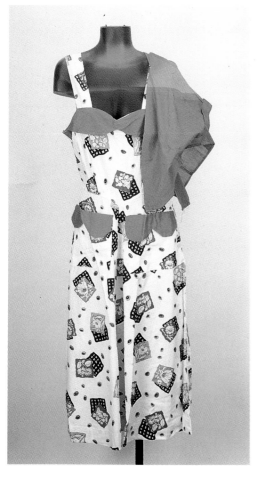

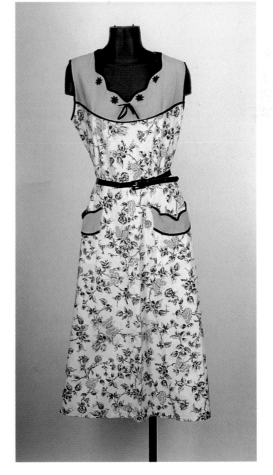

Sleeveless cotton sundress with matching bolero jacket, in a floral print with solid color trim, labeled Sue Sherry. $30-40

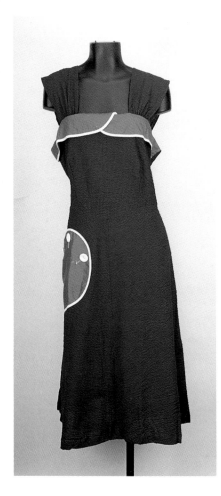

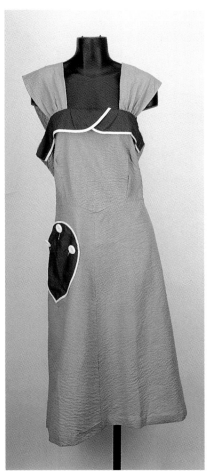

Identical sundresses made of crinkled cotton in different color combinations, labeled Fruit of the Loom. $25-35 each

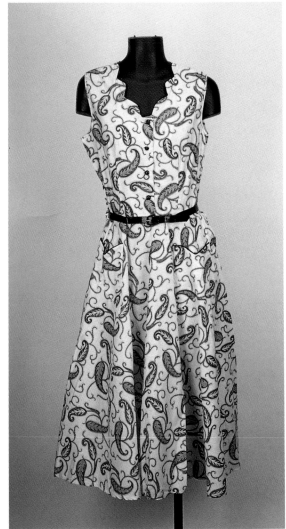

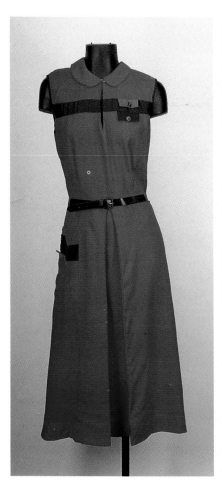

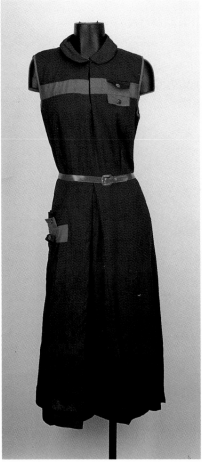

Sleeveless cotton dress with large paisley print, black trim, and a scalloped v-neckline, labeled Fruit of the Loom. $20-30

Two sleeveless rayon shirtwaist dresses with opposite color schemes, labeled Fruit of the Loom. $30-35 each

Suits

The thoroughly modern woman of the 1950s had many jobs, not only in the home, but out in the workplace. Besides wearing smart-looking dresses or slim skirts and blouses, the suit became the popular choice for the career-minded woman, especially those women wanting to climb the corporate ladder. With the advancement of synthetic fibers, the suit became easy to wear on and off the job.

The styles were numerous. Slim skirts were paired with fitted jackets. Boxy jackets teamed up with pleated skirts. Belted jackets looked great with straight skirts. Woven nubby checks, plaids and chevrons mated with rayon flannel. Similar to men's suitings, women's well-tailored suits were also made of wool flannels, tweeds and rayon pin stripes. Wool and Dacron teamed up quite often to create suits that were advertised as "crisp, fresh and carefree". Ads for suits made of DuPont Dacron in 1954 stated:

It's the look you love...from 9 till 5. No wonder so many busy women are finding "Dacron" polyester fiber the beautiful answer for work and play. They love its care-less ways — its delightful habit of keeping wrinkles at a minimum hanging into press overnight, saving inconvenient trips to the presser's.

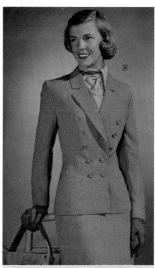

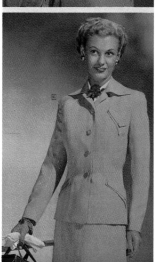

Two tailored suits made of gabardine advertised for sale in 1951.

Two piece navy and white tailored wool suit with decorative collar and pocket treatment, no label. $85-125

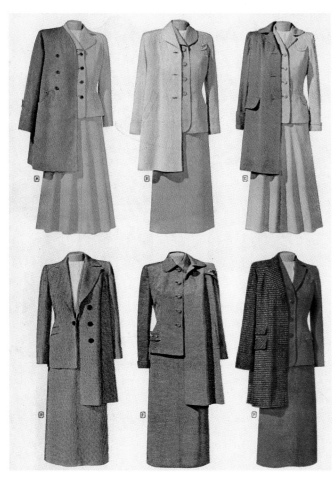

Ladies' suits and coordinating toppers in the popular colors and styles from 1953.

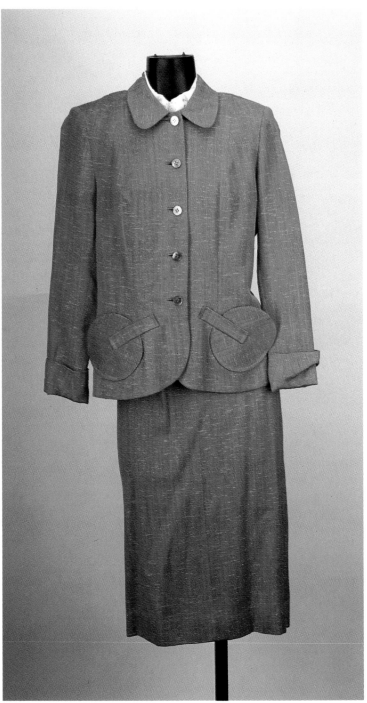

Mauve two-piece suit made of Rayon with Peter Pan collar, cuffs, and unsual pocket ornamentation, labeled Season Aire. $75-95

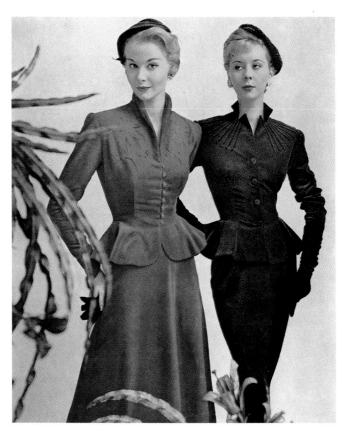

Two twill-back velveteen suits styled by Rose Bonazzi for Ronné Junior Dresses, New York, advertised in *Mademoiselle* in 1954.

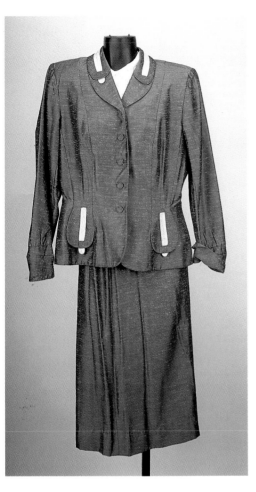

Two-piece gray silk suit with white braided trim on collar and pocket flaps, labeled Season Aire. $85-125

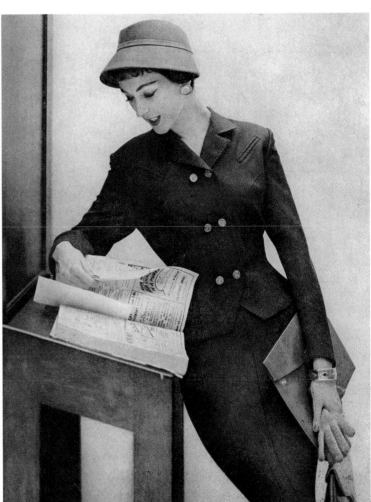

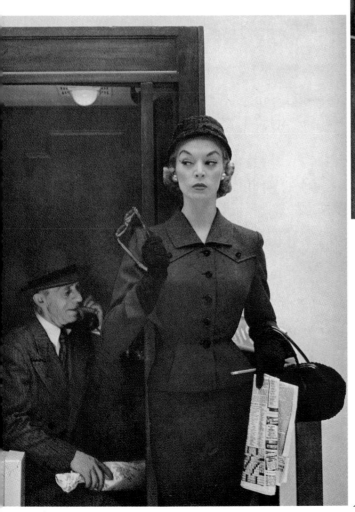

Ladies' suits for the executive types fashionable in 1954, advertised in *Charm*.

Circle Skirts

Circle skirts, made of yards and yards of fabric, entered the fashion scene in the late 1940s. The "Big Band" era coupled with the popular dance, the jitter bug, made the circle skirt on top of layers of crinolines the perfect attire. My mother told me many times of the poodle skirt she had custom-made for her in 1949. It was made of hot pink felt decorated with a black mink poodle and a rhinestone leash. Being an avid "jitter bugger", my mother had many circle skirts made for her in her dancing days. I wish she would have kept them! She never knew she'd have a daughter like me!

Some of the skirts from the late 1940s and into the early 1950s became very elaborate. Wool felt was extremely popular for poodle skirts, but poodles were not the only animals applied to circle skirts. Squirrels, kitty cats and other furry critters were found on 1950s felt circle skirts.

Flower themes were also popular design motifs for circle skirts. The look was achieved in many ways but the most desirable looks were done with silk screening, hand painting, flocking and embroidery. Rhinestones and sequins were also added for extra embellishment.

Circle skirts were usually worn with pullover sweaters, cardigan sweaters and sweater sets made of Orlon, virgin wool, angora and cashmere. Cute little blouses were also worn with circle skirts. Nylon, cotton, rayon and Dacron were the most popular fabrics used.

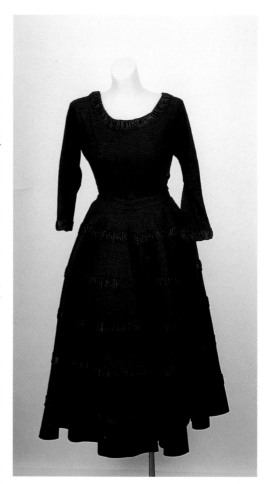

Two-piece outfit consisting of a black wool jersey top and black felt circle skirt, both accented with ribbon decoration. No label. $50-75

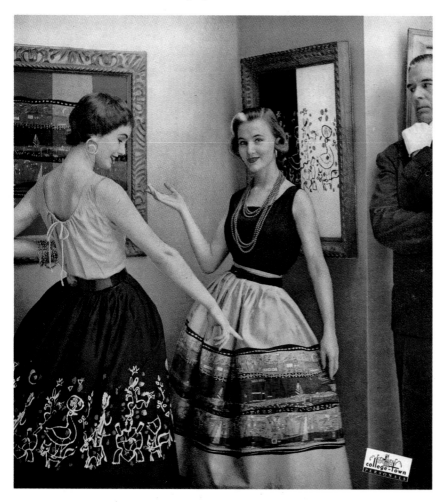

"Original Prints" by Lowenstein Signature Fine Art Fabrics made into circle skirts by leading designers and manufacturers. This was a popular trend in the mid-1950s.

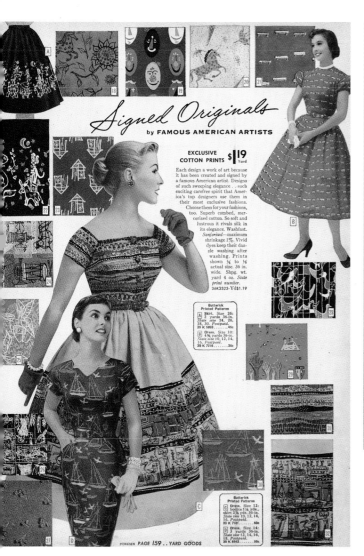

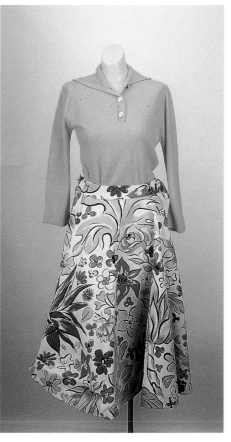

Heavyweight pink cotton circle skirt with exotic floral design. No label. $40-65
Salmon colored long sleeve pullover sweater made of Orlon, labeled Featherknits, "Look Sweeter in a Sweater, Nationally Advertised, Interlock Mazet Yarn by Milliken." $15-25

Signature fabrics became chic in the 1950s. This group of signed originals by famous American artists was offered for sale from Sears in 1955.

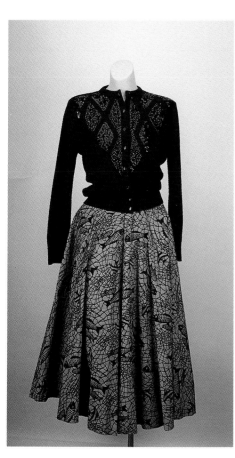

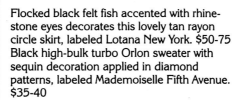

Flocked black felt fish accented with rhinestone eyes decorates this lovely tan rayon circle skirt, labeled Lotana New York. $50-75
Black high-bulk turbo Orlon sweater with sequin decoration applied in diamond patterns, labeled Mademoiselle Fifth Avenue. $35-40

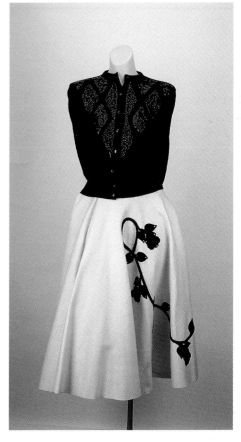

White felt circle skirt accented with stunning black velvet roses and rhinestone accents. No label. $50-75

25

A black and white denim-like fabric called sport denim makes up the body of this circle skirt, embellished with embroidery and accented with sequins. $50-75

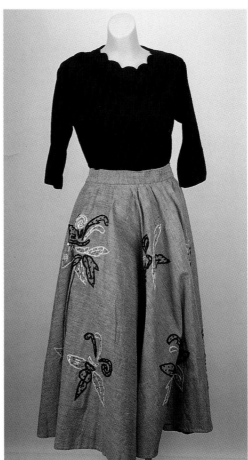

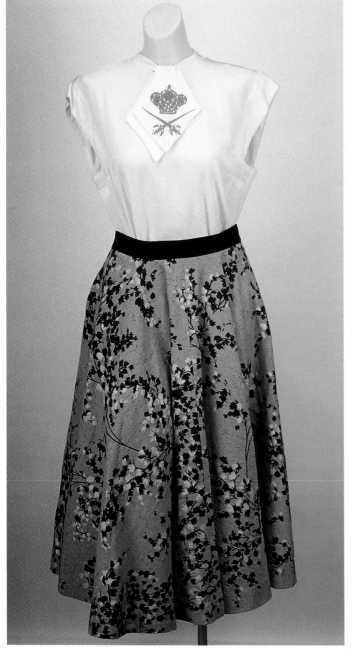

Circle skirt made of heavy weight cotton with hand printed floral decoration and velvet waistband, labeled Jo Collins. $40-60
White rayon blouse with cap sleeves, decorated with hand painted crown and sword motif accented with rhinestones. No label. $25-30

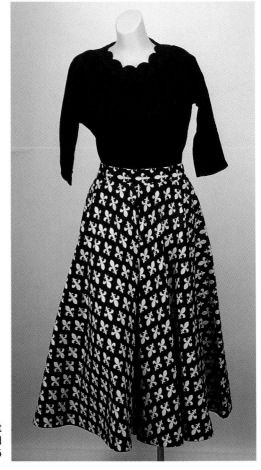

Black and white cotton circle skirt with *fleur-de-lis* pattern, labeled Modern Jr. $35-45

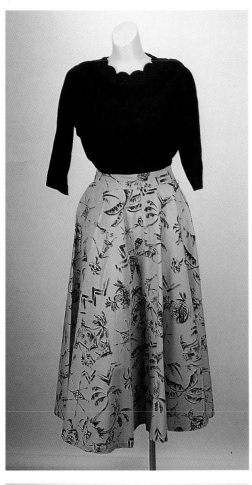

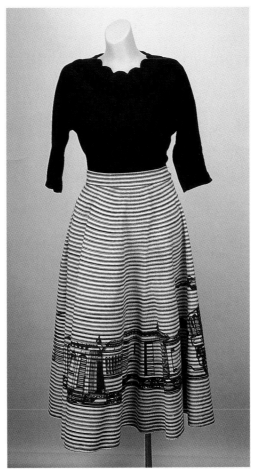

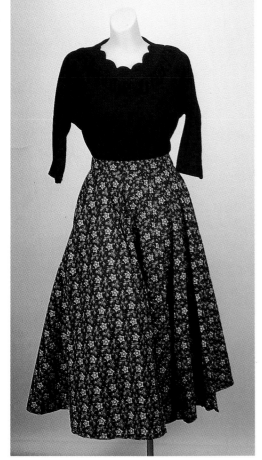

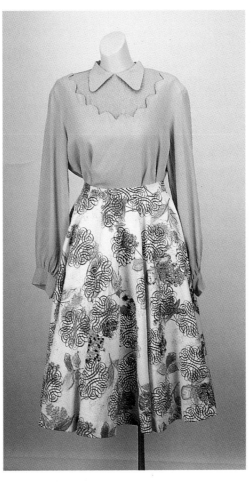

Top left: Light blue polished cotton circle skirt decorated with silk screened tropical print, labeled Fruit of the Loom. $35-45

Top right: Black and white horizontal striped circle skirt, with locomotive train design. No label. $45-65

Bottom left: Green and black floral printed cotton circle skirt, labeled A Willow Sportswear Original. $35-45

Bottom right: Long sleeve turquoise rayon crepe blouse with Peter Pan collar and pleated yoke, labeled A Mel Hahn & Gilbert Creation. $15-25
Circle skirt made of heavy weight cotton with hand printed floral decoration, accented with sequins. No label. $50-75

Textured cotton circle skirt with silk screened floral and animal print. No label. $40-50
Polished cotton short sleeve blouse with rounded neckline accented with rhinestones, labeled Cotton Cutie by Harwill. $20-25

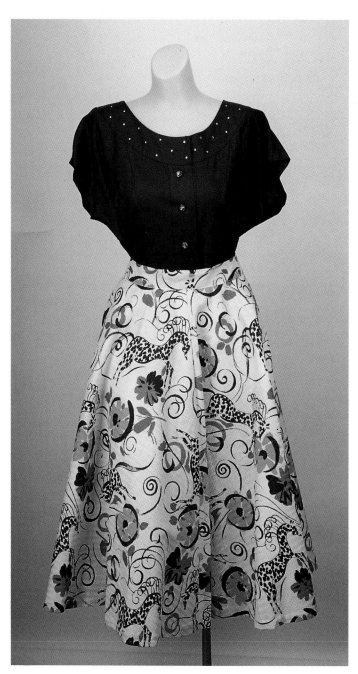

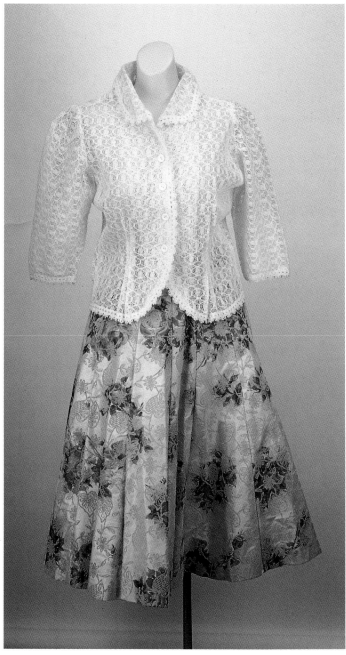

Beautiful polished cotton circle skirt with hand printed floral decoration and flocked leaf designs. No label. $45-65
Button down lace top made of cotton, with Peter Pan collar. No label.

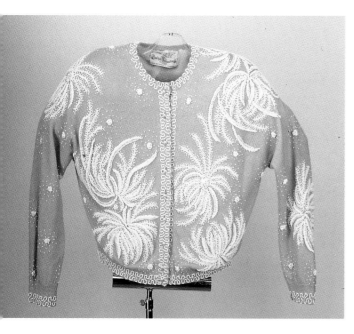

Cardigan sweater made of lambs wool, angora, and nylon, decorated with milk glass beads applied in a palm tree design, labeled Boutique International, California-Hand decorated in Hong Kong. $45-60

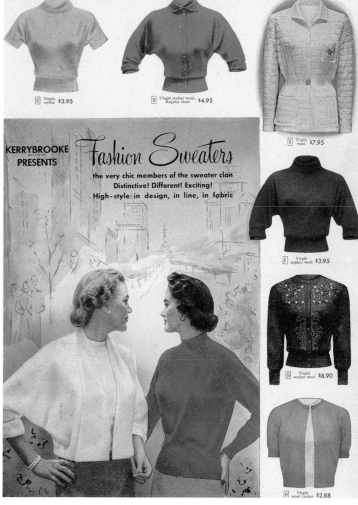

"Kerrybrooke" brand sweaters, made of Virgin wool and Nylon, were offered for sale from Sears, Roebuck & Company in 1953.

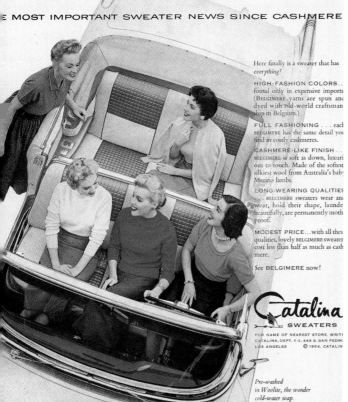

"Catalina" brand sweaters made of Belgimere, an Australian lamb's wool, were advertised in *Charm* magazine in 1954.

Casual Wear

The casual look for women of the 1950s consisted of Capri-pants, pedal pushers, Bermuda shorts, knit tops and halter tops. Many of the casual styles which were advertised in period magazines and catalogs were described as "Italian-Inspired" or "In the Italian Manner" largely due to the fact that many of these new looks were actually first seen in Italy and the island of Capri and designed by Italian designers.

The styles eventually made there way to America. With the dawning of the "Jet Age" travel became a world-wide pastime. Casual clothing was being advertised with the tourist in mind. For example, assorted colors of sport denim, made into Capri pants, Bermuda shorts, pedal pushers, circle skirts, halter tops and visor caps were advertised as "California-Styled". For the exotic-minded, a long jacket with belted waist, labeled the "Jamaica Jacket" made of poplin came in many colors like Matador Red, Mexican Orange or Bahama Blue. Not only was the clothing itself given an exotic name, but the color of the garment as well. All of these merchandising techniques helped to generate sales, and made casual clothing a 1950s phenomenon.

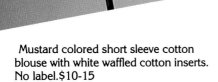

Mustard colored short sleeve cotton blouse with white waffled cotton inserts. No label.$10-15

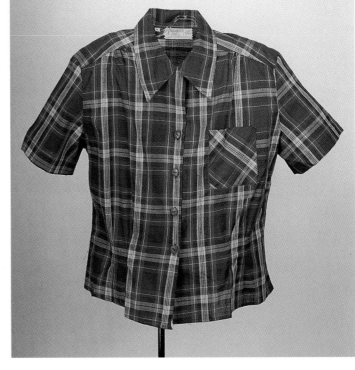

Short sleeve cotton blouse with plaid design, labeled Tailortex Classic, A US Royal Fabric, United States Company. Original tag reads: United States Rubber Company Presents Yarmouth Gingham, One of the New US Royal Fabrics. $10-15

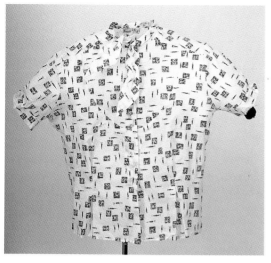

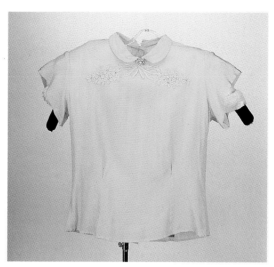

Mustard colored rayon crepe blouse with Peter Pan collar and floral appliques studded with rhinestones. No label. $20-30

Short sleeve blouse made of Dacron with abstract print, labeled Winnie Kaye. $10-15

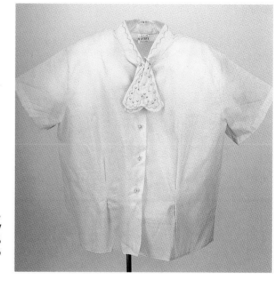

Pink short sleeve blouse, accented with embroidery and beadwork, labeled 100% Dupont Dacron. $18-25

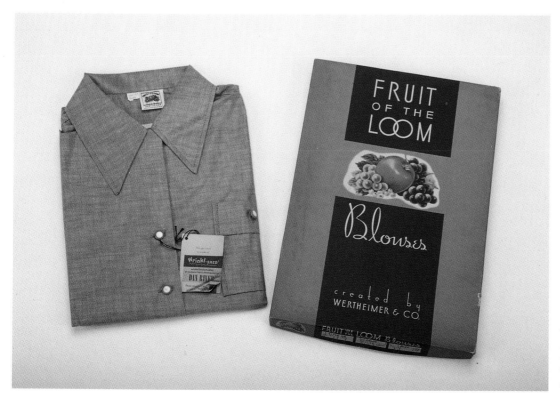

Lady's blouse made of denim-like polished cotton with decorative buttons, labeled Fruit of the Loom created by Wertheimer & Co. Presented with its original box. $15-20

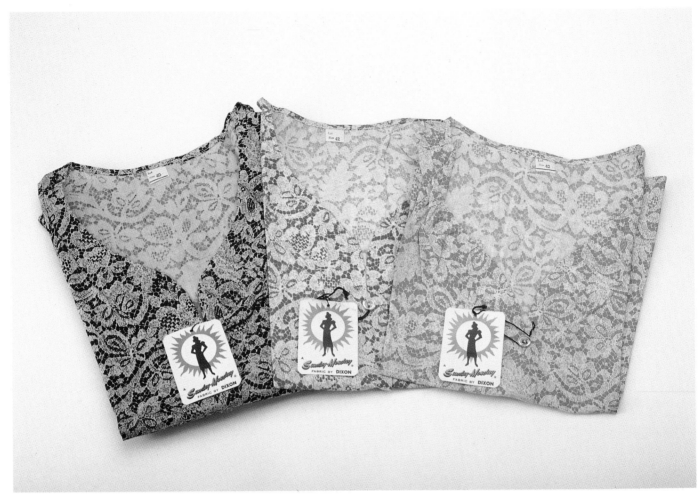

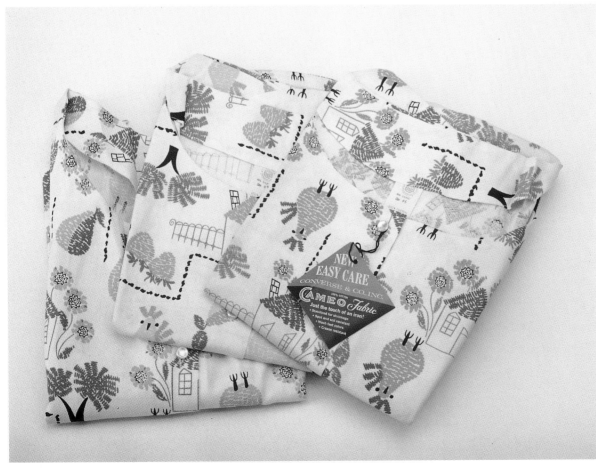

Three, lady's blouses made of cotton with a printed lace pattern in assorted colors. The tag reads "A Sunday-Monday Fabric by Dixon." $10-15

Trio of textured cotton blouses with colorful summer prints. The tag reads 100% Cameo Fabric, Just the Touch of an iron! $10-15 each

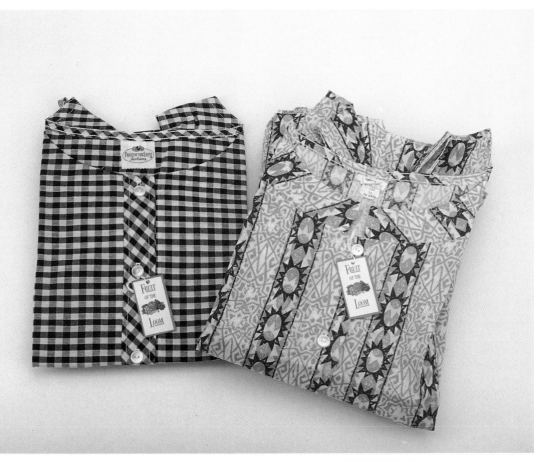

Two, sleeveless, cotton, summer blouses with checked and abstract prints, made by Fruit of the Loom. $10-15 each

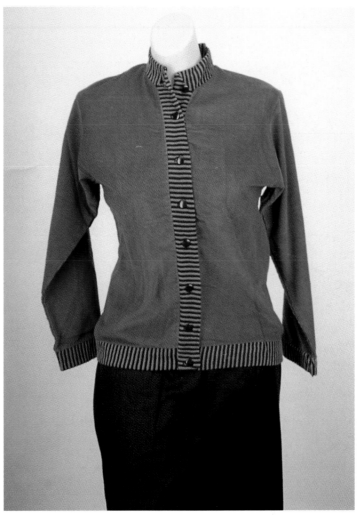

Rust colored long sleeve corduroy blouse, accented with black stripes, labeled Arlene Originals. $15-20

33

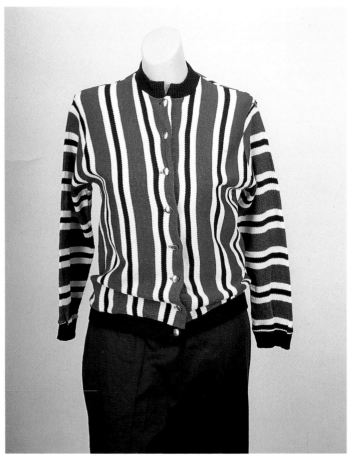

Vertical striped, long sleeve top made in a three-toned color combination, accented with gold tone buttons, and solid color collar and waistband, labeled Arlene Originals. $15-20

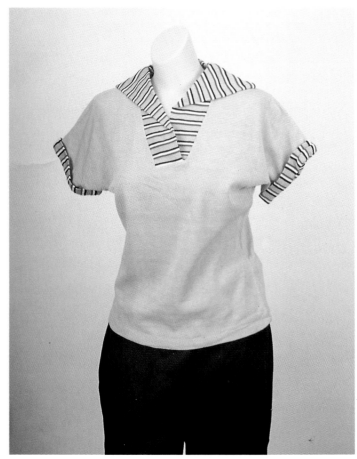

Short sleeve beige knit top decorated with red, white and black striped trim, labeled Arlene Originals. $12-18

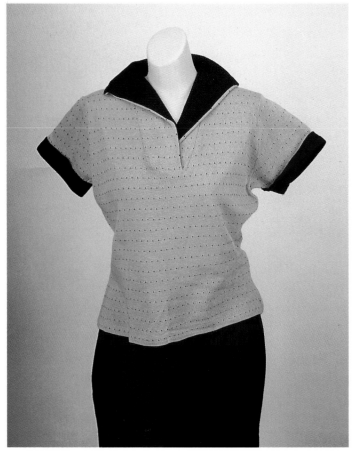

These mix & match denim separates, made in bright colors, were offered for sale from Sears in 1955.

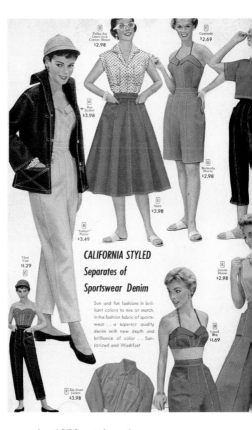

An Arlene Original in the popular 1950s pink and black color combination. $15-20

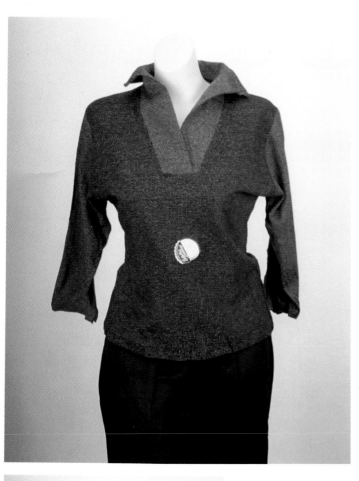

Black cotton capri pants, labeled Fruit of the Loom; another Arlene Original Knit top in black and rust. $15-25

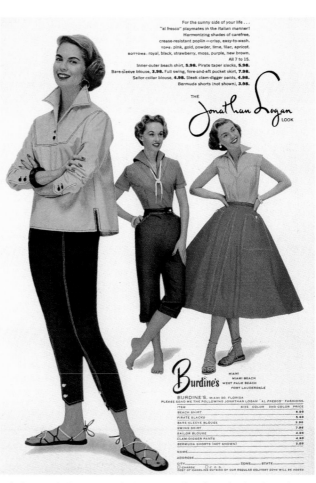

Italian-styled summer fashions made of poplin by Jonathan Logan in 1955.

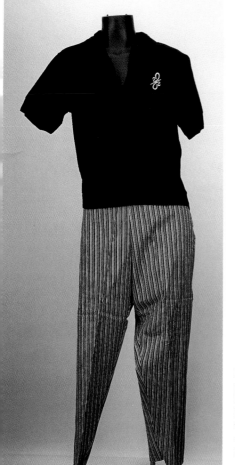

Plaid Bermuda shorts, pedal pushers and slacks made of a rayon fiber called "Coloray", advertised in the Fall of 1954.

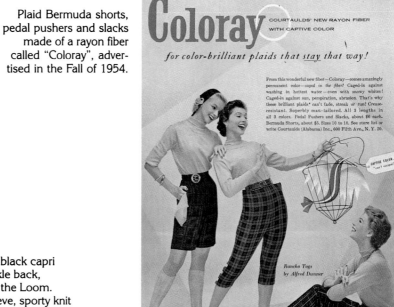

Red, white and black capri pants with buckle back, labeled Fruit of the Loom. Black short sleeve, sporty knit top with V-neck and white embroidered decoration, labeled Andrea. $10-20 each

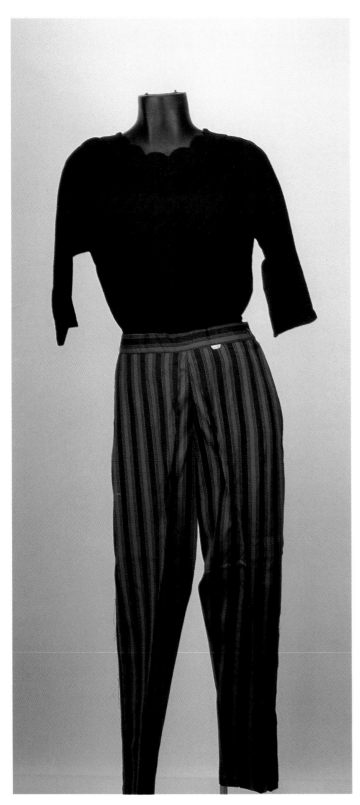

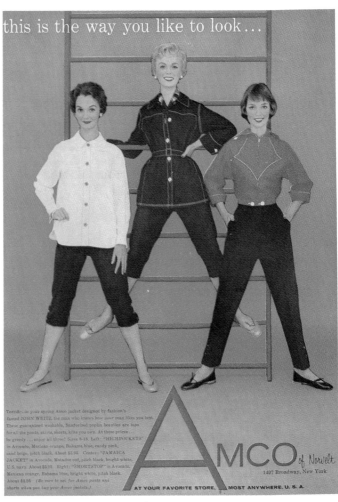

Sporty poplin fashions designed by John Weitz and featured in *Charm* magazine in 1955.

Brown and black striped capri pants with buckle back.
No label. $15-25
Black jersey knit pullover top with scalloped neckline. No
label. $10-15

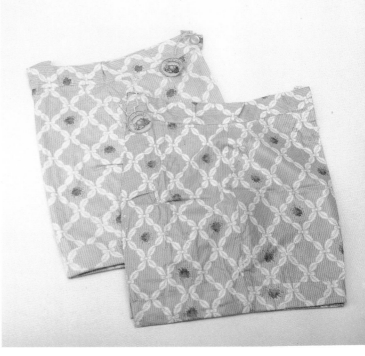

Two pair of lady's shorts made of polished
cotton with pretty floral print by Fruit of the
Loom. $8-12 each

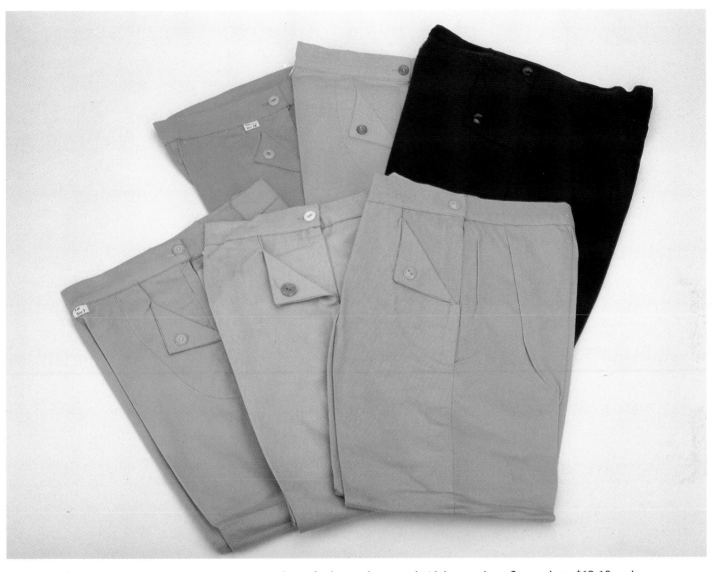

Six pair of ribbed cotton capri pants in a rainbow of colors and accented with button-down flap pockets. $12-18 each

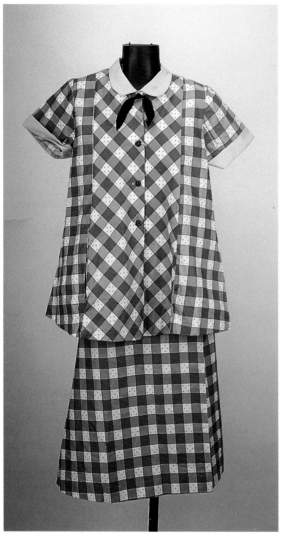

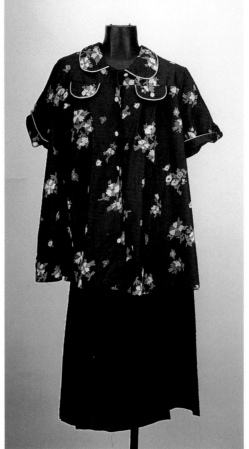

Two-piece maternity outfit consisting of solid black skirt and floral printed smock top, labeled Fruit of the Loom Maternity. $30-40

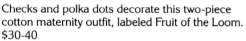

Checks and polka dots decorate this two-piece cotton maternity outfit, labeled Fruit of the Loom. $30-40

In the 1950s, clothing for Mothers-To-Be was made a little differently than it is today. Maternity skirts or pants, usually part of a two-piece ensemble, were made in one of two ways. The options were either a "Cut-out" front, whereas a circular section of the fabric was actually cut-out allowing for growth, or a "zip-to-fit" waistband making the garment adjustable as needed. Smart jackets and smock tops were paired up with the skirts and pants creating neat and stylish looks for the pregnant women.

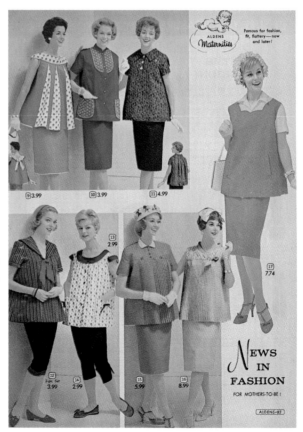

Colorful maternity fashions for "Mothers-To-Be" offered for sale in 1959 from Aldens.

Two-piece maternity outfit of cotton with scenic printed smock top and solid black skirt, labeled Fruit of the Loom Maternity. $30-40

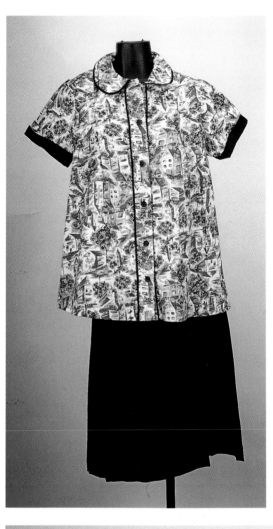

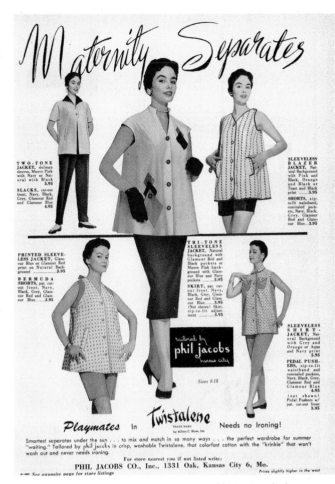

Maternity clothes tailored by Phil Jacobs of Kansas City in 1955.

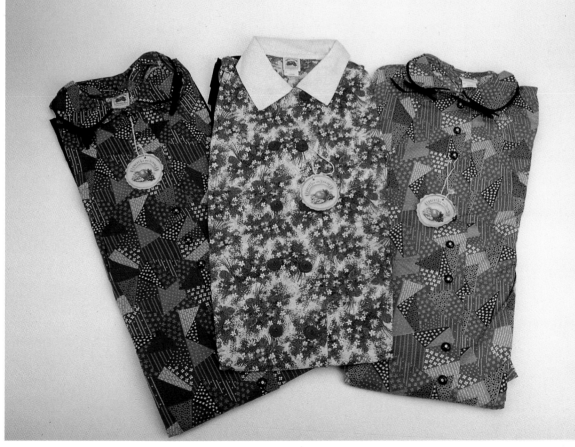

Three lady's maternity sets consisting of black cotton skirts and printed cotton tops, labeled Fruit of the Loom. $30-40 each

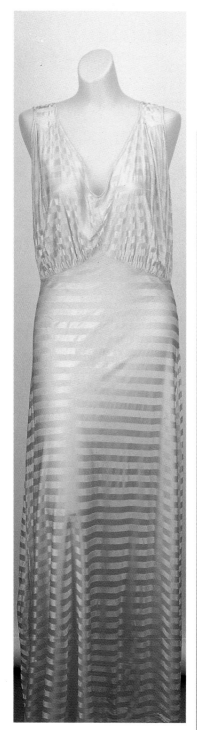

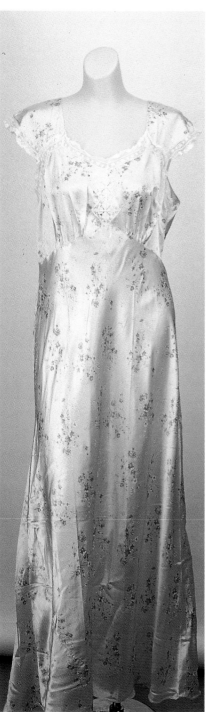

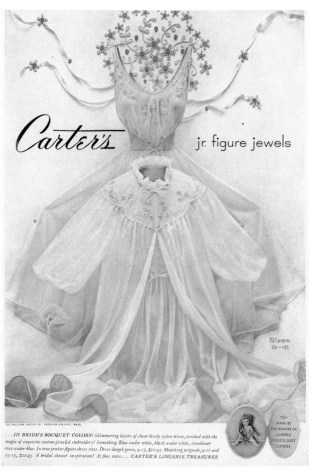

Carter's Nylon tricot lingerie accented with jeweled embroidery advertised in *Mademoiselle* in 1954.

Sleeveless nightgown made of peach colored banded nylon, labeled Van Raalte. $25-30

Rayon nightgown with floral print, trimmed in off-white lace. No label. $25-35

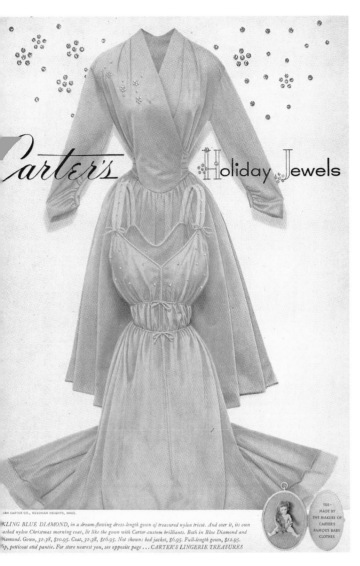

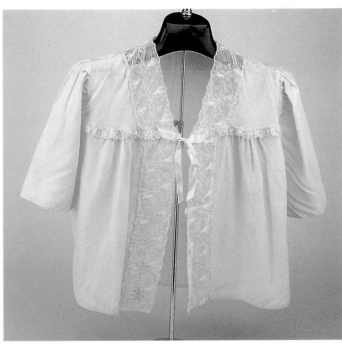

Lady's, pink nylon bed jacket with embroidered tricot trim and pink ribbon tie closure, no label. $15-20

Lovely ladies' nightgown and matching robe made of Nylon tricot by Carter's, featured in *Charm* magazine in December of 1954.

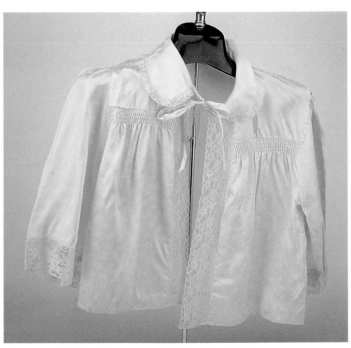

Lady's, pink Rayon bed jacket with lace trim and ribbon closure, no label. $20-25

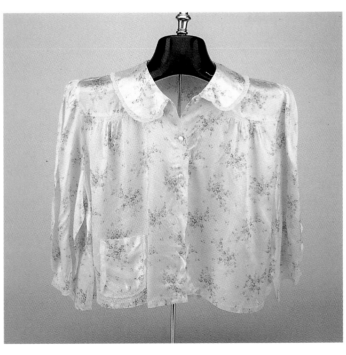

Lady's, white print Rayon bed jacket with pearl buttons and lace trim, no label. $20-25

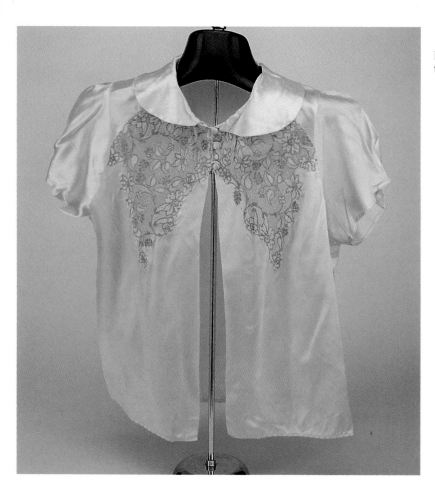

Lady's, pink Rayon bed jacket with purple lace trim and three fabric covered buttons, no label. $20-25

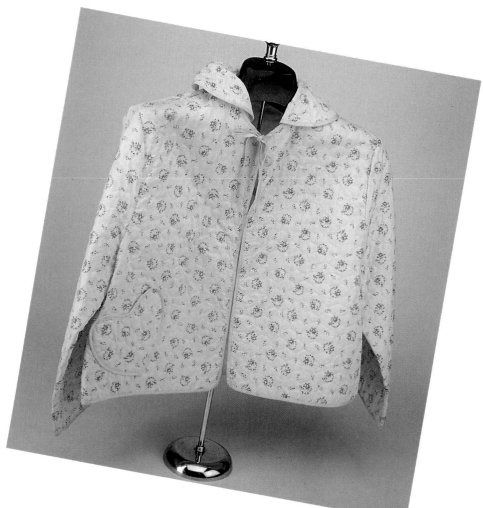

Lady's, yellow print, quilted bed jacket, no label. $18-25

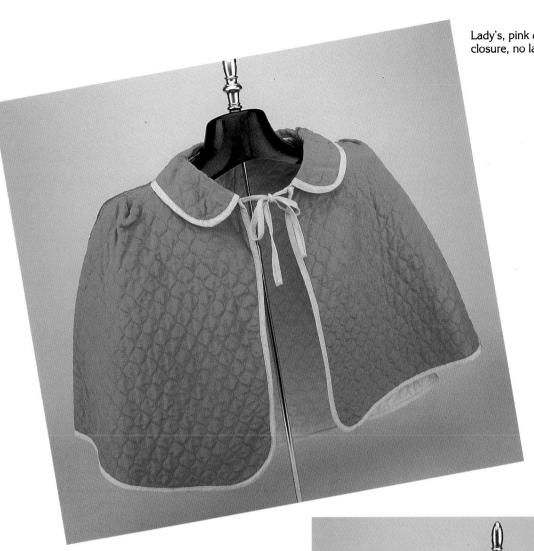

Lady's, pink quilted bed cape with tie closure, no label. $20-25

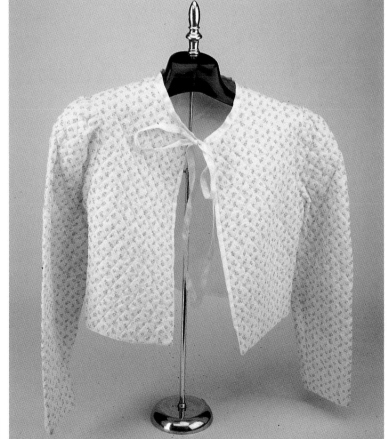

Lady's, yellow print, quilted bed jacket with white tie closure, no label. $15-20

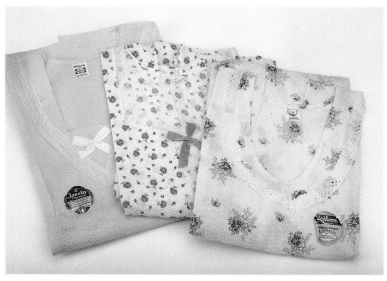

An assortment of solid color and printed lady's crinkle cotton night-gowns trimmed with nylon and cotton lace, labeled Artloom, Helen Joan, and Wash-an-redy. $15-20 each

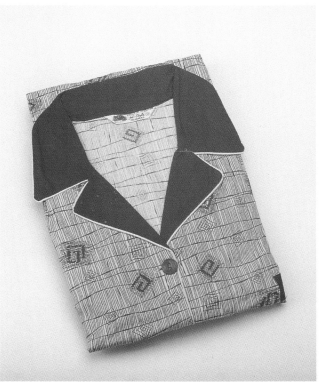

Tailored pajamas made of red and white cotton with an abstract print and solid color collar, labeled Fruit of the Loom Hi-style Pajamas. $25-35

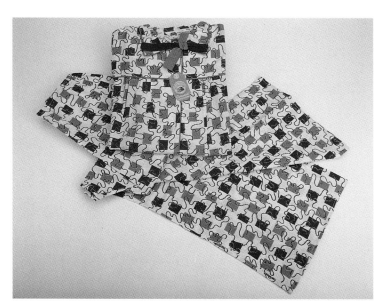

Lady's cotton print pajamas, labeled Fruit of the Loom Hi-Style Pajamas. $15-20

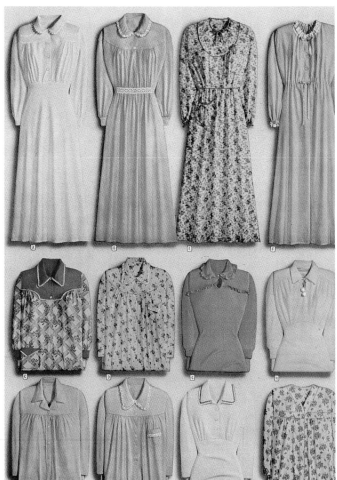

Flannette nightgowns and pajamas in solid colors and prints from 1950.

44

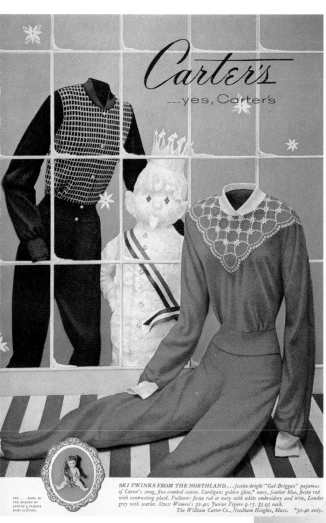

Ladies' ski pajamas by Carter's, "Makers of Carter's Famous Baby Clothes", August, 1954, *Charm*.

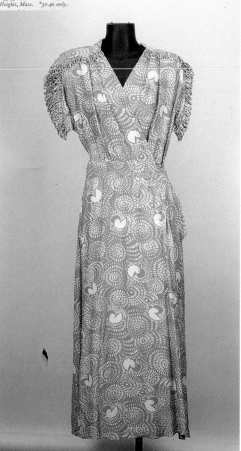

Chenille housecoat and lounging robes made of rayon and cotton in flattering styles from 1950.

Bottom left: Lovely blue rayon lounging robe with floral print, no label. $35-45

Bottom center: Lounging robe made of turquoise and white rayon with an abstract print, accented with loop decoration, labeled Textron. $35-45

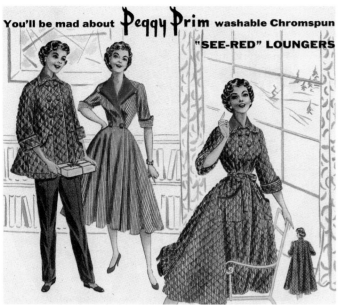

You'll be mad about **Peggy Prim** washable Chromspun "SEE-RED" LOUNGERS

Quilted pajamas, shortie robe and duster, all trimmed in red velvet by "Peggy Prim," advertised for the Christmas holiday season in 1954.

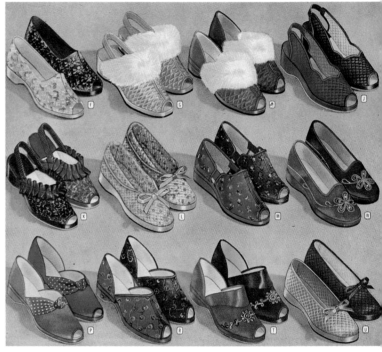

Ladies' slippers designed for "at-home leisure" shown here in the popular styles and colors from 1950.

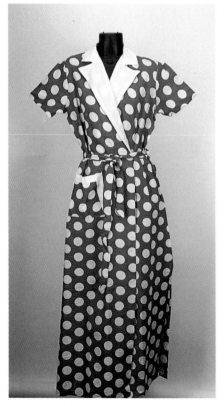

Crinkled cotton lounging robe with large polka dot print, in teal and white, labeled Blondette. $30-35

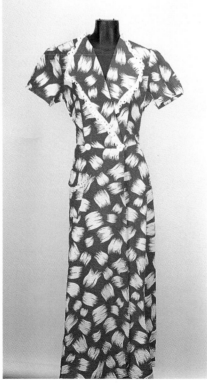

Crinkled cotton lounging robe with red and white brush stroke pattern, trimmed in cotton eyelet, no label. $30-35

Lingerie

Fashions designed for night wear in the 1950s was a broad category consisting of nightgowns made of rayon, nylon and satin, many lavishly trimmed in lace or embroidery. Satin-striped rayon was extremely fashionable in the early part of the decade usually offered in peach, pink or light blue. Pretty bias-cut gowns with Empire waists were made of solid-color or floral printed fabric. The designs were stylish and extremely flattering. The gowns were available with matching robes or bed jackets.

Nightgowns and pajamas were also made of crinkle cotton, cotton percale, acetate tricot, broadcloth, rayon crepe, rayon jersey, flannel and assorted blends.

Loungewear for at-home leisure consisted of long robes, short robes, brunch coats and pajamas. Quilted cotton, seersucker, rayon, cotton plisse and chenille were the popular fabrics used throughout the decade.

Slips

A large percentage of the ladies' slips that were offered for sale throughout the 1950s were as beautifully designed as the nightgowns of that era. Rayon crepe and rayon satin were popular and advertised as…"a most luxurious lingerie fabric that lends itself beautifully to a graceful fit". Nylon was also extremely popular and noted for its easy laundering and quick drying qualities.

Whole slips were trimmed in exquisite lace, fancy eyelet and ruffles. They were also embroidered or applied with appliqués. The most common colors were pink, peach, light blue, navy, yellow, Nile green, black and white. Cotton slips were also common, attractively styled and moderately priced.

Crinolines or bouffant petticoats were extremely desirable especially for the fashions that required that extra fullness. Made of materials like nylon net, nylon taffeta, acetate taffeta, nylon parchment taffeta and nylon horsehair, these cancans were flirtatiously frilly and a must for full-skirted fashions.

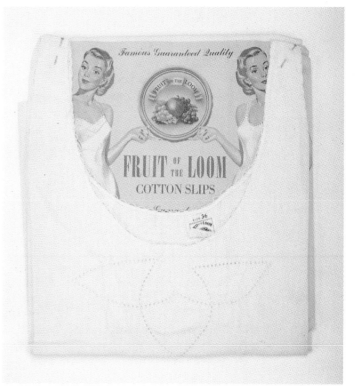

Cotton full slip with an openwork pattern and edging added for decoration, labeled Fruit of the Loom. $3-6

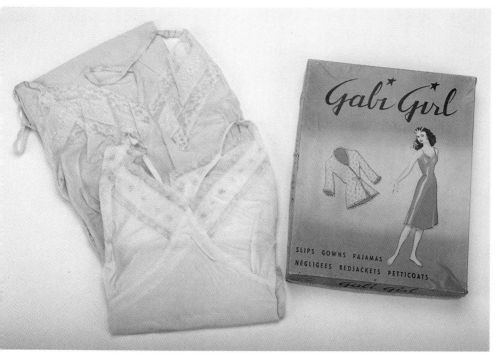

Nylon slips with lace trim and embroidered decoration, accompanied by their original box, labeled Styled by Gabi Girl. $4-8 each

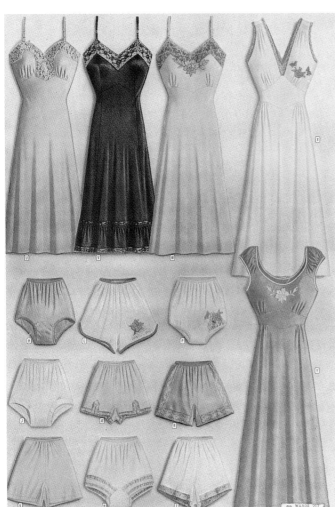

Nylon slips, nighties and panties offered for sale from Montgomery Ward in 1950.

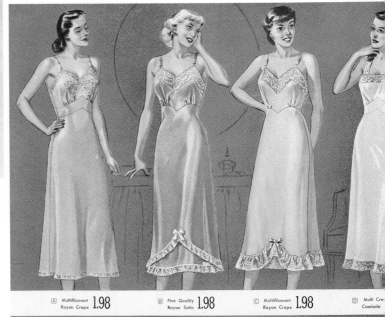

[A] Multifilament Rayon Crepe 1.98	[B] Fine Quality Rayon Satin 1.98	[C] Multifilament Rayon Crepe 1.98	[D] Multi Crepe Camisole

Colorful slips made of rayon crepe and satin accented with ribbon and lace offered for sale in 1950.

[E] Multifilament Rayon Crepe 2.98	[G] Multi Crepe Godet Slip 2.98	[H] Satin Elegant with Lace 2.98	[J] High Style Multi Crepe

48

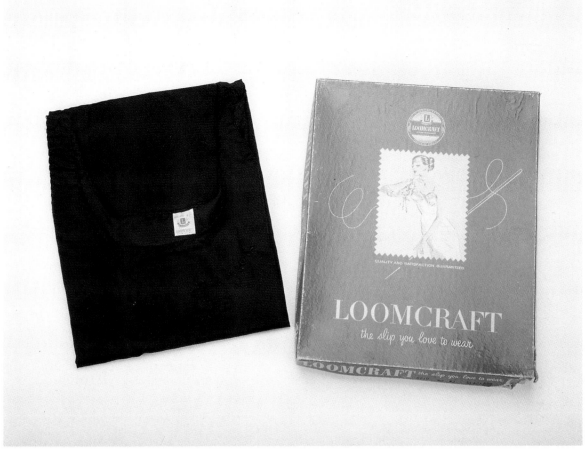

Lady's slip made of black acetate with embroidered decorations, accompanied by their original box, labeled Loomcraft Styled Loveliness. $4-8

Lady's slip made of plain white cotton accompanied by its original box, labeled Lingerie by Velrose, Softer, Smoother, Longer Lasting. $5-10

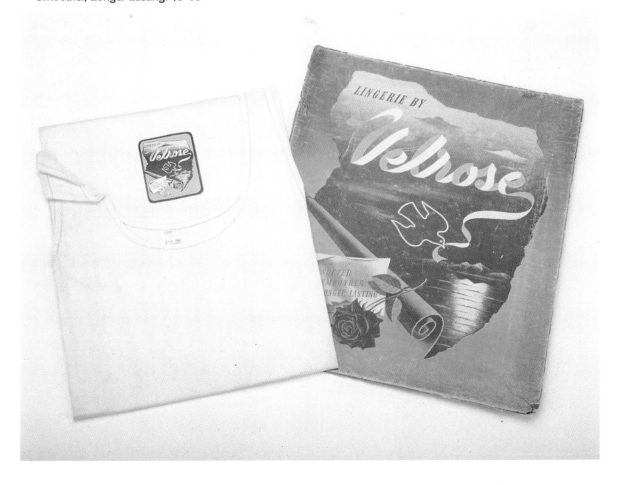

Foundation Garments

Fashionably speaking, bras and girdles were the necessary foundation garments worn by the woman of the 1950s. Bras made by well-known manufacturers combined "flattery with practical wear" and provided a "definite uplift and support for a flattering bust line".

In 1955, the "curvallure" bra by Jantzen was described as "the wonderful new glamorizer, best padded bra ever designed...to fill out your bust line, give your figure rhythm, make your clothes fit better, look better...naturally, comfortably, gracefully".

Bras designed with circular-stitched cups were sometimes referred to as "whirlpool" bras which provided a comfortable lift. This type of bra was extremely popular in the mid-1950s when fashion terminology, "the high bosom look" was used. Today, this type of bra is sometimes referred to as a bullet bra.

Longline bras were also popular and described as being worn to control the diaphragm and provide support. They were worn to slim and smooth the waistline without boning, as was common in corsets.

Girdles were a must for the fashion conscious woman of the 1950s, not to mention that pantyhose did not enter the fashion scene yet. Numerous girdle styles were offered for sale through mail-order catalogs all predicting to mold one's figure or provide "figure flattery". Some girdles gave adequate control while others offered to give firm control. For all-over control, one-piece corsets and corselets were offered, some even designed with coil wire boning for "control plus comfort". The all-in-one corset or girdle was especially designed for the long-torso look because it molded the body curves from shoulder to thighs.

Corselets were "designed to smooth out all your figure problems at one sweep, with front and rear panels to keep both views in good form".

For the gal with the heavier figure, girdles and one-piece corsets were designed with inner belts for "special abdominal support" or front and back laced corsets for "excellent abdominal control and firm back support".

For women with full, pendulous abdomens, some girdles were advertised as "scientifically designed posture aids "with a front panel firmly boned to improve the appearance. Maternity girdles were also common for the pregnant woman. Girdle styles were endless. In one Sears, Roebuck & Company mail-order catalog from 1953, girdles were featured on twenty-five pages.

Bras and Girdles

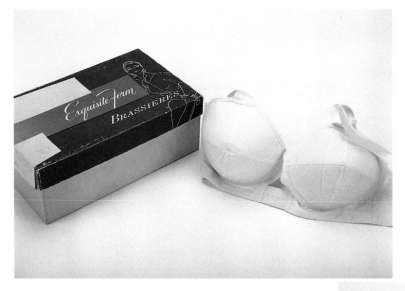

Cotton bras with their original box, labeled Exquisite Form Brassieres Circle-O-Form. $8-10 each

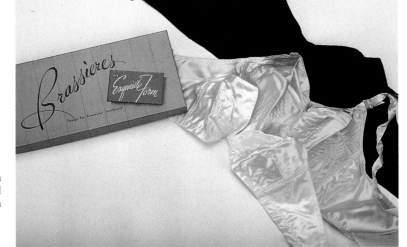

Assortment of Exquisite Form satin bras in white, black, and pink. $6-12 each

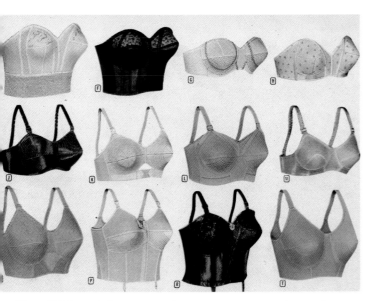

The 1955 line of "Joan Browne" bras in regular, strapless and long line designs.

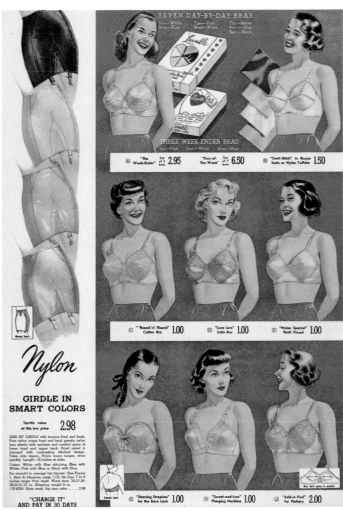

Popular styles in ladies' bras and girdles offered through mail-order in 1950.

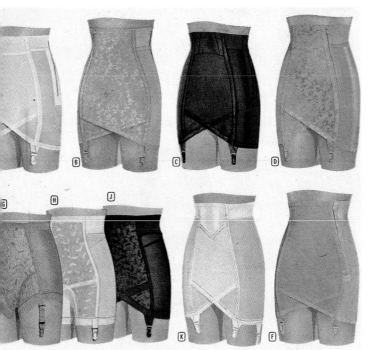

"Sarong" girdles made of Nylon taffeta, rayon and cotton batiste, Nylon mesh and rayon and cotton brocade in the popular styles from 1955.

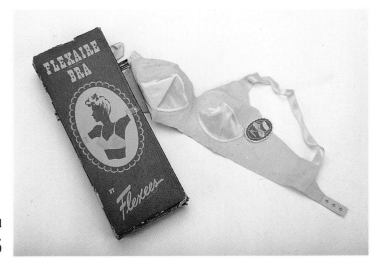

Peach-colored bra made of rayon and cotton, shown with its original box, labeled Flexaire Bra by Flexees. $5-10

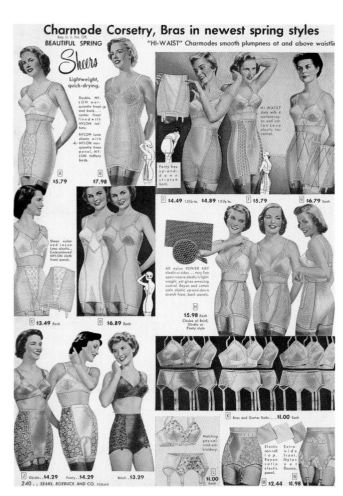

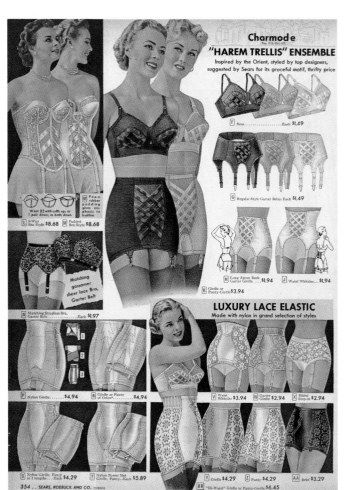

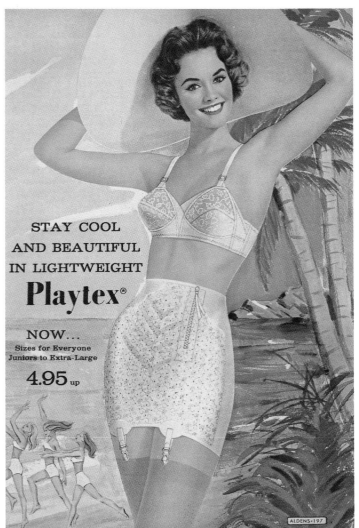

"Charmode" brand corsets, bras, girdles and garter belts offered for sale from Sears in 1951.

An advertisement for "Playtex" bras and girdles featured in the Aldens catalog in the Summer of 1959.

Bras, girdles and garter belts in fashionable styles and colors from 1953 featured in the Sears mail-order catalog.

Hosiery

Besides girdles being worn for figure flattery, they were also necessary for holding up the seamed and seamless Nylon stockings of this era. Stocking were like the icing on the cake; they became the focal point to form a complete and glamorous look from hem line to shoe. They flattered the legs and the sheerer, the better.

Nylon hosiery was offered for sale in many price ranges depending on the quality and sheerness of the nylon. Determining the sheerness was dependent upon the denier and the gauge. The denier represented the nylon yarn size; a low count means a sheer nylon. The gauge, on the other hand, refers to the number of stitches or the number of needles used in knitting the stocking. For example, 15 denier, 51 gauge is an ultra sheer stocking designed for evening wear, while a 70 denier, 45 gauge nylon is service weight and designed for heavy-duty wear.

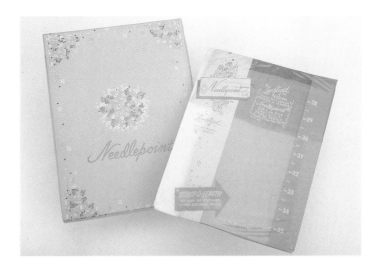

Following eight photos: Group of nylon stockings, several with interesting heel and seam designs in contrasting colors. The paper boxes are printed with stylish packaging designs. Labels and box names include Fruit of the Loom, Lady Barbara, Bamrose, Elaine Arden, Celtic Maid, Quaker Maid, Lady Ronalda, Miss Thrifty, and others. $3-15 pair

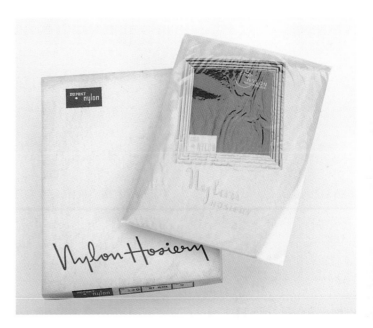

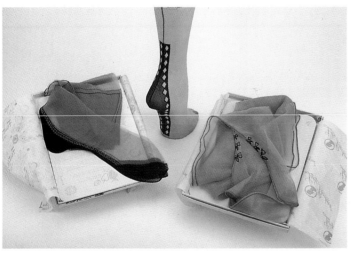

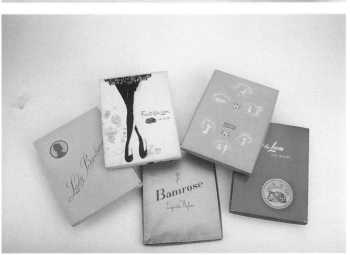

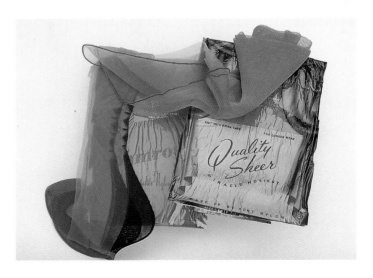

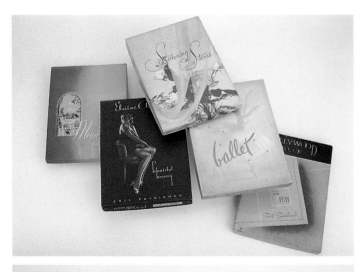

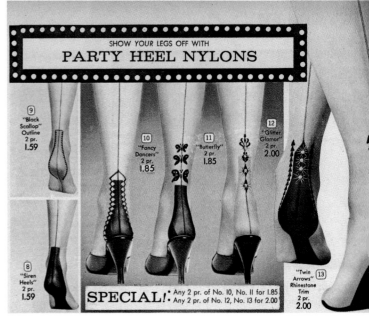

Seamed stockings with extra embellishment at the heel -a classy look popular in the late 1950s.

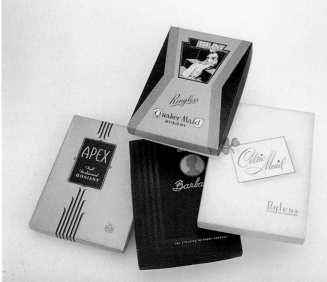

"CAREFREE" Nylons in four leg-flattering colors offered from Sears, Roebuck and Company in 1951.

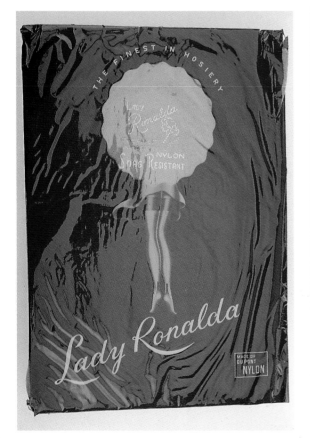

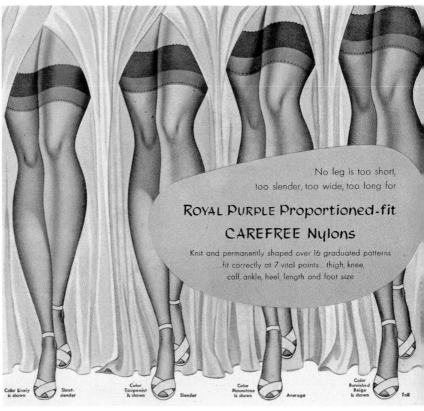

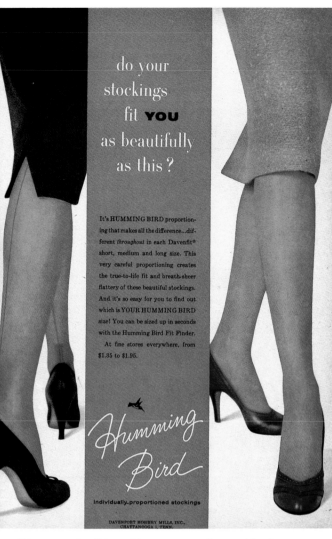

do your
stockings
fit **YOU**
as beautifully
as this?

It's HUMMING BIRD proportioning that makes all the difference...different *throughout* in each Davenfit® short, medium and long size. This very careful proportioning creates the true-to-life fit and breath-sheer flattery of these beautiful stockings. And it's so easy for you to find out which is YOUR HUMMING BIRD size! You can be sized up in seconds with the Humming Bird Fit Finder.

At fine stores everywhere, from $1.35 to $1.95.

Humming Bird

individually-proportioned stockings

DAVENPORT HOSIERY MILLS, INC.,
CHATTANOOGA 1, TENN.

"Humming Bird" brand hosiery manufactured by Davenport Hosiery Mills advertised in *Charm*, March, 1955.

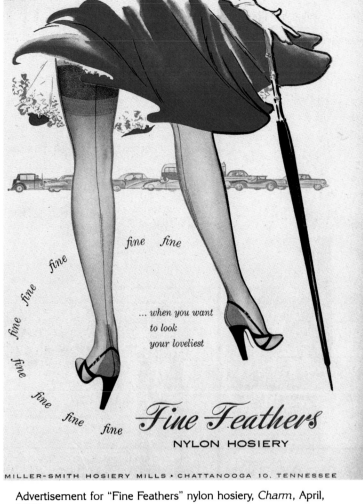

fine fine fine fine fine fine fine fine fine fine

... when you want
to look
your loveliest

Fine Feathers
NYLON HOSIERY

MILLER-SMITH HOSIERY MILLS · CHATTANOOGA 10, TENNESSEE

Advertisement for "Fine Feathers" nylon hosiery, *Charm*, April, 1955.

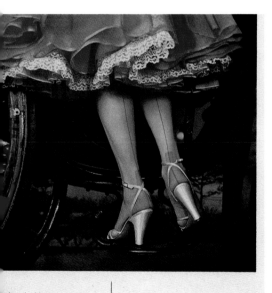

Seamed nylon stockings manufactured by DuPont and advertised in *Charm* in 1955.

nal touch of beauty
... hosiery of

Du Pont Nylon

To the tip of your toes . . . you look your loveliest . . . thanks to today's more-beautiful-than-ever nylons! Right now, the stores are ready with brand-new nylons . . . in unbelievable sheers and lovely weights for busy days. Treat yourself to a wardrobe of nylon hosiery in the colors and weights of spring!

DU PONT
BETTER THINGS FOR BETTER LIVING
...THROUGH CHEMISTRY

xciting new things are happening in **NYLON** — one of **DU PONT'S** modern-living fibers

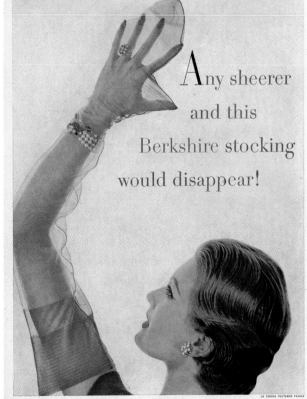

A ny sheerer
and this
Berkshire stocking
would disappear!

These are full-fashioned 10 denier nylons, the sheerest stocking you can buy. And because Berkshire makes them, you'll find they offer you the same dependable Nylace Top and Toe-Ring protection against runs that start from top or toe, as the Berkshires you buy for every day. Proportion-knit, of course. sheer sheer **BERKSHIRE** STOCKINGS

"Berkshire" ultra-sheer seamed stockings, a popular brand of nylon hosiery offered for sale in the 1950s.

Shoes

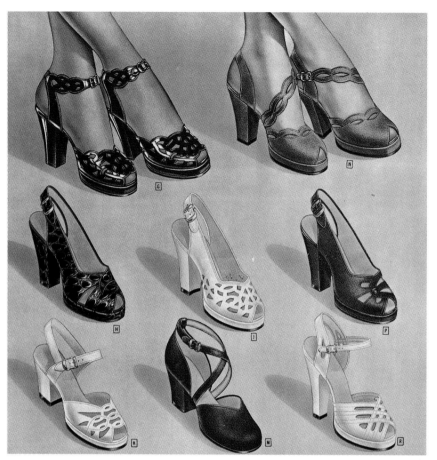

Classy styles in ladies' sandals and pumps offered for sale in 1950.

Opposite page:
Top left: This lovely assortment of ladies' shoes in fashionable colors was offered for sale from Montgomery Ward in 1955.

Top right and bottom right: This extremely colorful array of ladies' shoes and sandals was offered for sale from Spiegel in 1950.

Bottom left: Advertised as "This year's College Headliners", these shoes for young women were popular in 1955 and advertised for sale from Montgomery Ward.

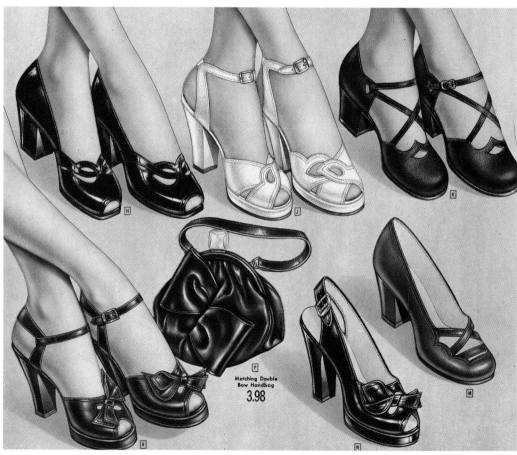

Matching Double
Bow Handbag
3.98

Fine quality leather pumps advertised in Spiegel in 1950.

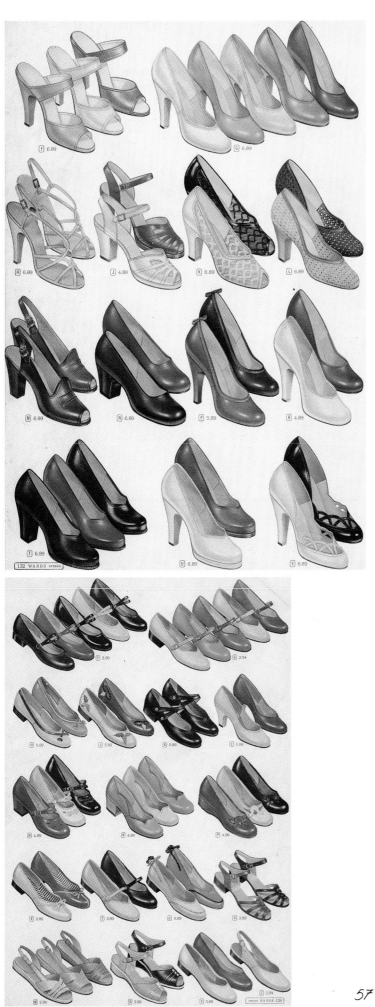

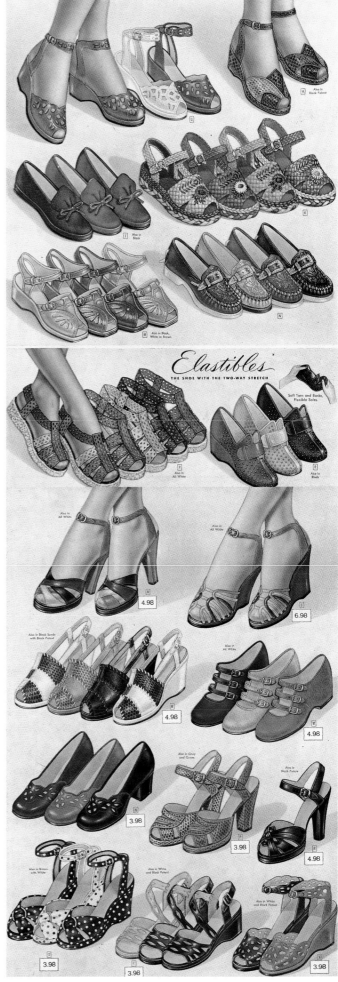

Accessories

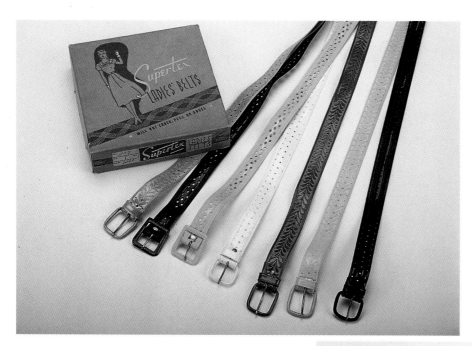

Assortment of vinyl belts for ladies in a rainbow of colors accompanied by their original box, labeled Supertex. $3-5 each

Three, lady's, organdy and printed polished cotton aprons with waist ties, not labeled. $4-8 each

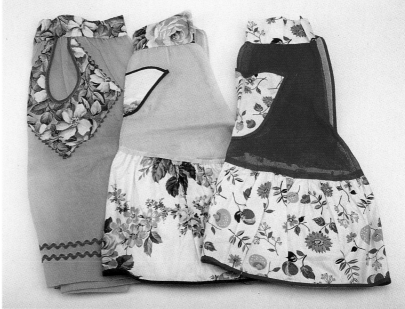

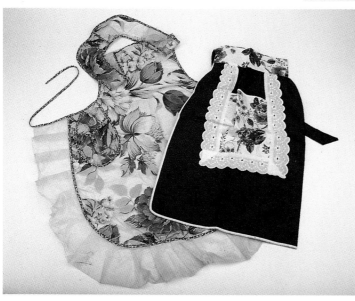

Two, lady's aprons, one made of textured cotton with floral printed pockets accented with rhinestones trimmed with white eyelet, and the other one of printed flexible plastic with bib top and waist ties, not labeled. $4-8 each

Chapter 11
Fashions for Young Women & Girls

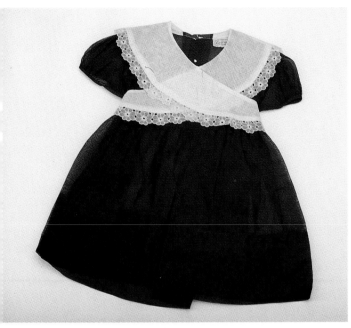

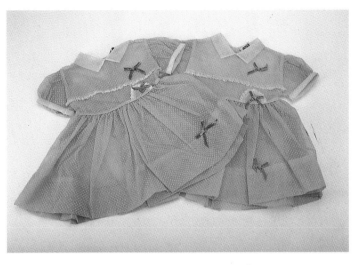

Two, nylon, dotted Swiss girl's dresses trimmed with lace and velvet, labeled Tiny Town Togs. $12-18 each

Navy blue and white organdy dress with lace trim labeled La Ronda, Fashions For Girls. $12-18

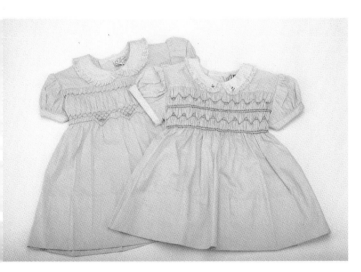

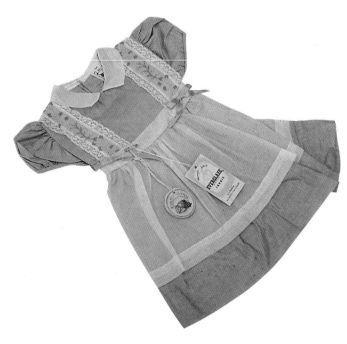

Pink and yellow cotton dresses with white collars and cuffs, decorated with smocking and embroidery. $15-20

Little girl's, blue, party dress with a white organdy apron attached, labeled Fruit of the Loom. $12-18

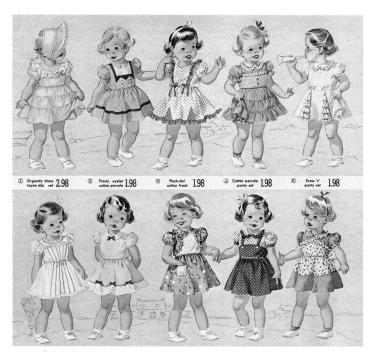

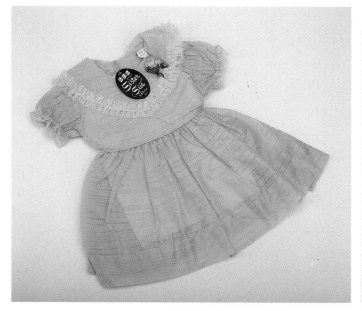

Dresses for "Tiny Tots" accented with ruffles, eyelet, dainty dots and ribbon featured in Spiegel in 1950.

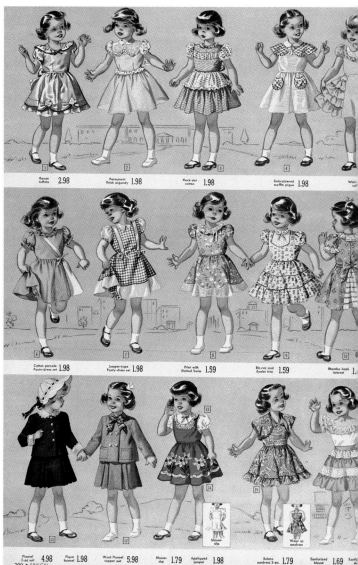

Adorable dresses and ensembles for little girls made of organdy, rayon taffeta, wool flannel and cotton in the popular styles from 1950.

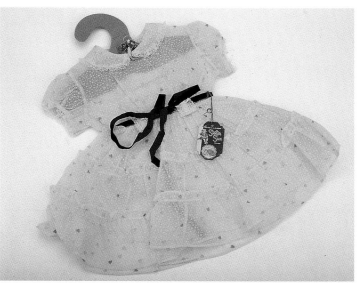

Little girl's, pink, party dress with white lace trim, labeled Fruit of the Loom Sister Sue Frock. $15-20

Little girl's, printed, yellow organdy dress with black velvet waist ribbon, labeled Fruit of the Loom Sister Sue Frock. $15-20

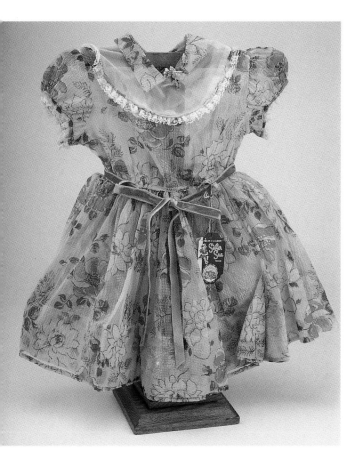

Little girl's floral printed party dress of textured nylon with blue velvet waist ribbon, labeled A Fruit of the Loom Sister Sue Frock. $15-20

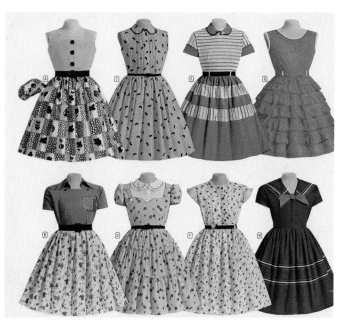

Advertised as "Smart Styles for Sizes 7 to 14", these cute dresses made of cotton and nylon were stylish in 1955.

Two, little girl's, party dresses of sheer nylon with satin waist ribbons, labeled A Fruit of the Loom Sister Sue Frock. $15-20

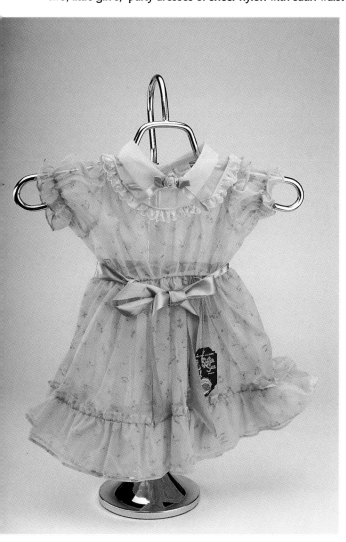

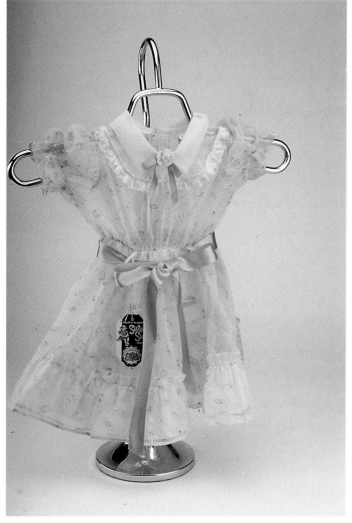

Girl's, green and yellow textured cotton, summer pinafore, labeled Winsome Frock. $12-18

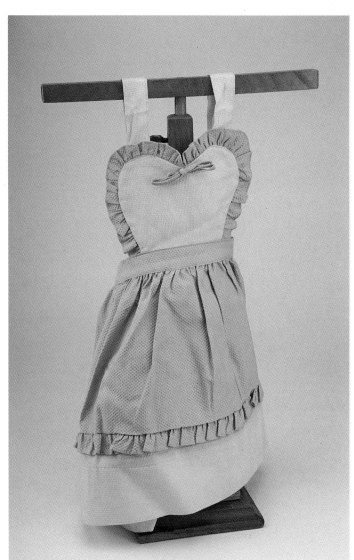

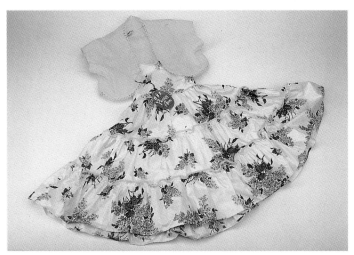

Girl's, polished cotton print sun dress and matching yellow bolero jacket, labeled Peggy Ann Frocks. $15-20

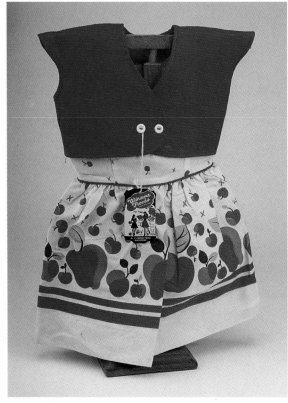

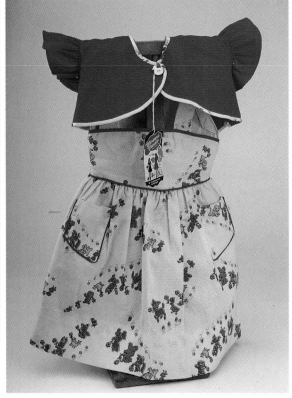

Two, girl's, cotton print sundresses and matching red bolero jackets, labeled Winsome Frock. $15-20 each

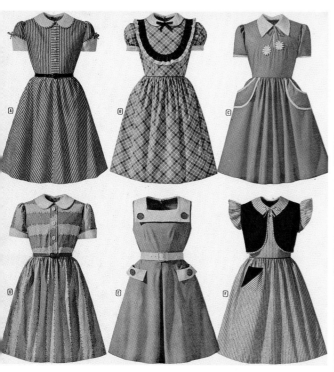

Cotton dresses for young girls in assorted styles and prints fashionable in 1953.

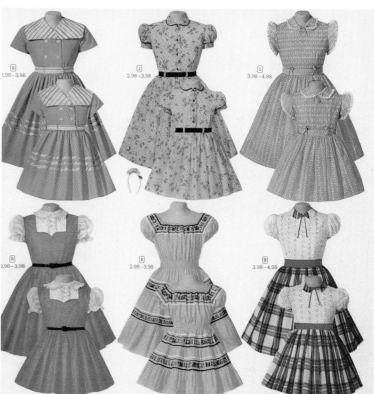

Sister dresses in assorted styles from 1955 made of embossed cotton, puckered nylon, flocked nylon and embroidered eyelet.

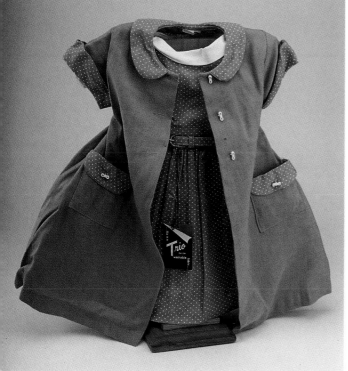

Girl's, blue, rayon dress and matching coat with white trim, labeled Sister Sue. $20-25 set

Matching dresses for "Mother and Daughter" made of Twistalene - "a crinkle cotton that needs no ironing", *Charm*, April, 1955.

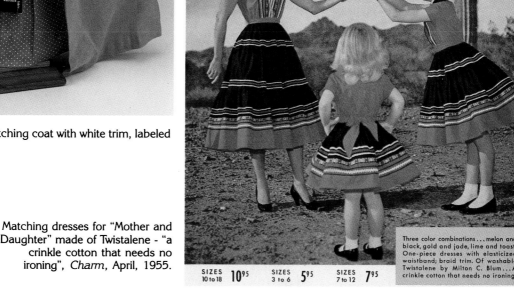

Patio Fashions!
A trio in *Twistalene®* by
SUN RAY OF
ARIZONA

| SIZES 10 to 18 | 10⁹⁵ | SIZES 3 to 6 | 5⁹⁵ | SIZES 7 to 12 | 7⁹⁵ |

Three color combinations...melon and black, gold and jade, lime and toast. One-piece dresses with elasticized waistband; braid trim. Of washable Twistalene by Milton C. Blum...A crinkle cotton that needs no ironing.

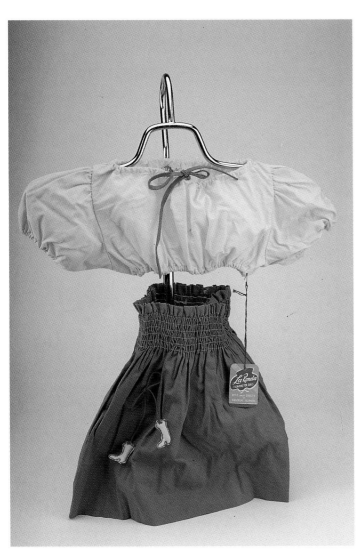

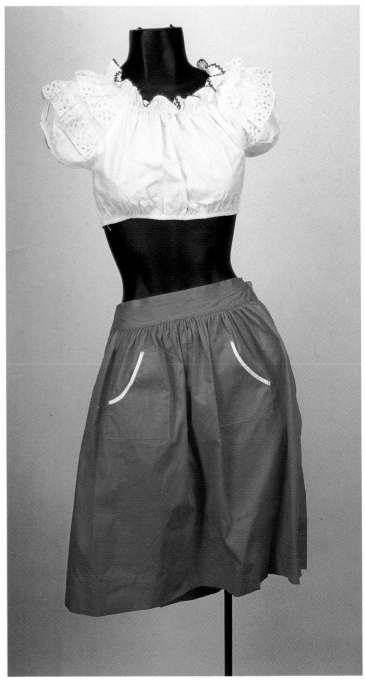

Girl's, two-piece, cotton outfit with yellow peasant-style top and brown skirt ornamented with a tie and dangling cowboy boots, labeled LaRonda Fashions for Girls. $12-18

Young lady's two-piece outfit made of cotton consisting of a full skirt and peasant blouse trimmed with cotton eyelet and rick-rack, blouse labeled Phyl-Mor Frocks. $12-18

Blouses

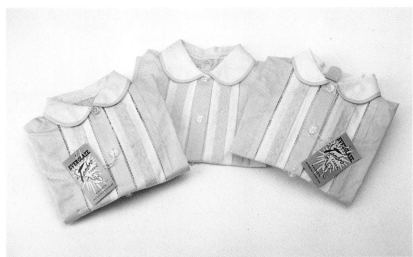

Trio of blouses in assorted colors made of washable Everglaze, a durable wrinkle and soil resistant fabric by Tanbro. $7-10 each

Two little girl's blouses made of cotton with Peter Pan collars, puffy sleeves, and lace trim, labeled A Chippy Original. $8-10 each

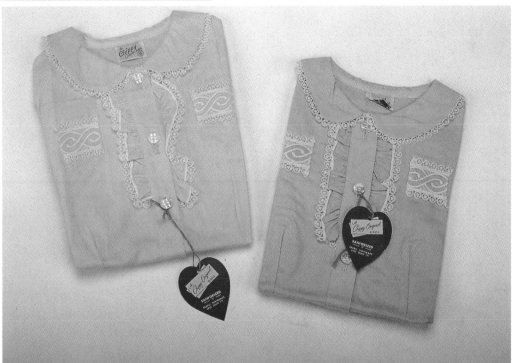

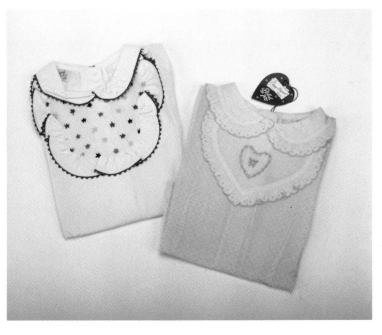

Two little girl's blouses with puffy sleeves and Peter Pan collars, trimmed with rick rack and fancy edging, both accented with embroidery, labeled A Chippy Original. $8-10 each

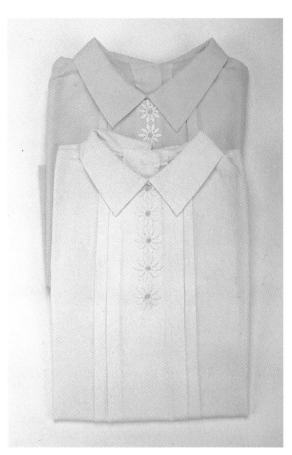

Two little girl's blouses made of textured cotton with floral appliques, labeled A Chippy Original. $6-10 each

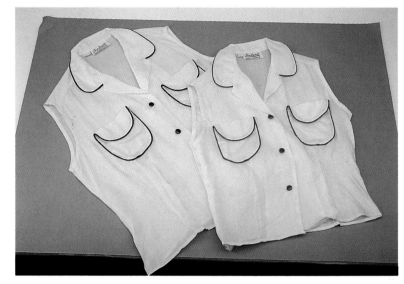

Two, girl's, white sleeveless cotton blouses with colored piping and buttons, labeled Jack Daniels by Wertheimer & Co. $5-10 each

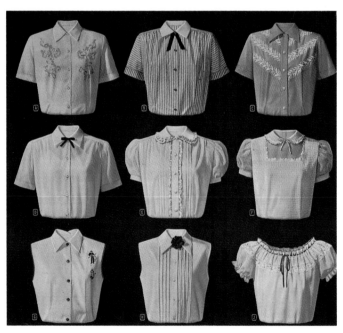

Blouses for young girls made of nylon crepe, cotton broadcloth and acetate and nylon in assorted styles fashionable in 1953.

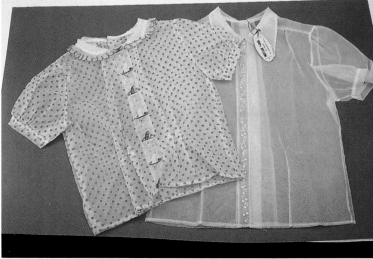

Two, girl's, nylon blouses, one with red dots and Mexican hats embroidered down the front, and the other with embroidered pastel flowers, labeled Kitty Kollier. $8-12 each

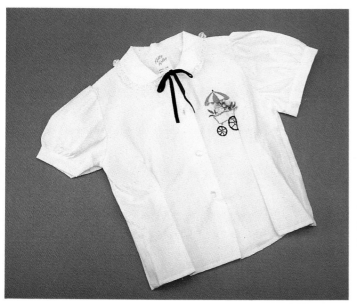

Girl's, white, ribbed cotton blouse with embroidered flower cart decoration, labeled Kitty Kollier. $8-12

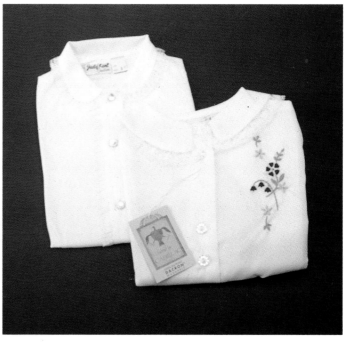

Two white blouses made of Dacron, decorated with embroidery. The Peter Pan collars are trimmed with nylon lace, labeled Judy Kent Creation. $6-10 each

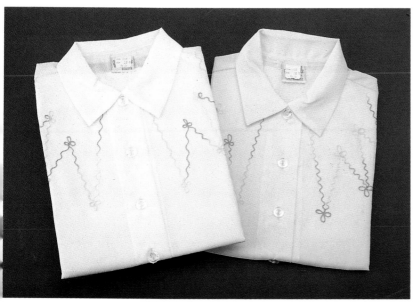

Identical blouses made of pink and white Dacron and accented with embroidery, labeled Betty Winkel. $6-10 each

Identical blouses in different color combinations made of drip-dry cotton with Persian print, labeled Betty Winkle. $5-10 each

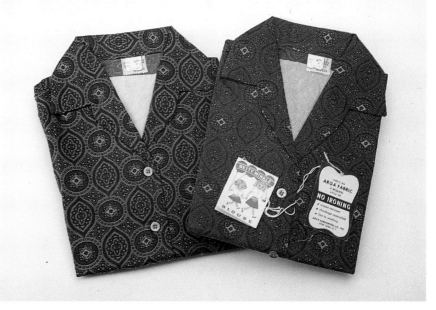

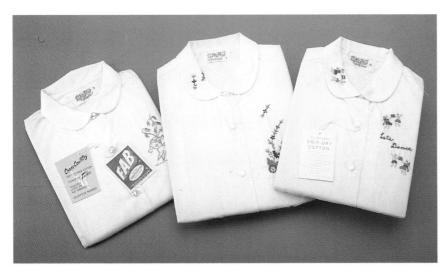

Three, combed cotton blouses with Peter Pan collars and embellished with embroidery, labeled Jo-Jo by Judy Kent. $8-12 each

White Dacron blouse designed with Peter Pan collar, short puffy sleeves, and silk screened print of a lady with a poodle, labeled Judy Kent creation. $8-12

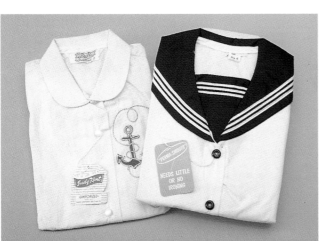

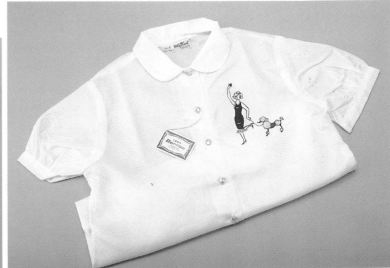

Two, white cotton blouses, one with blue and white sailor collar, the other with an anchor and braid decoration, labeled Jo Jo by Judy Kent. $7-10 each

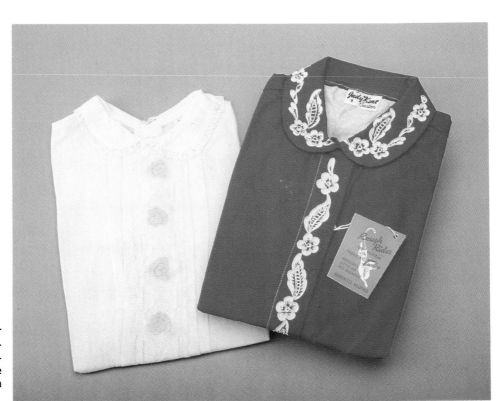

Red cotton blouse with Peter Pan collar decorated with silk edging and hand-painted flowers, labeled Judy Kent. Off-white organdy blouse trimmed with lace and labeled A Chippy Original. $8-12 each

Sweaters

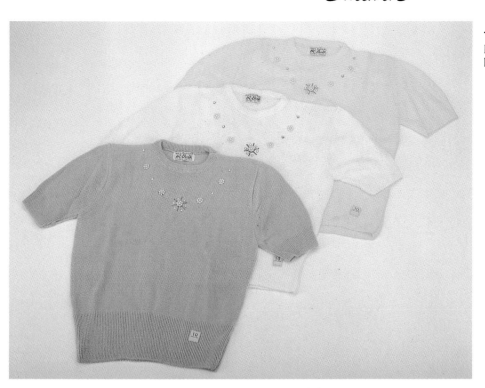

Trio of girl's pullover sweaters made of Hi-Bulk super Orlon and embellished with beadwork. $12-18 each

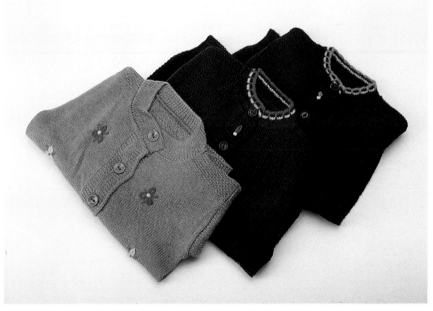

Three, girl's button-down cardigan sweaters made of wool and accented with embroidery. $6-12 each

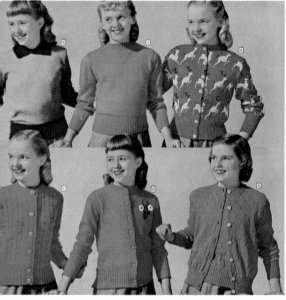

Little girls' sweaters made of wool and nylon designed in pullover and cardigan styles from 1950.

Skirts

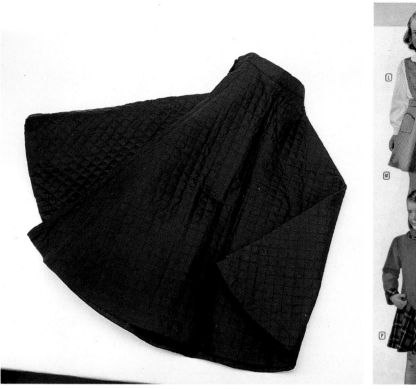

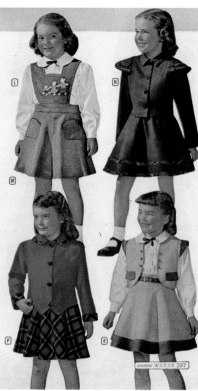

Girls' jumpers and suits made of wool, flannel and corduroy offered for sale from Montgomery Ward in 1950.

Girl's, dark blue, quilted circle skirt, no label. $18-22

Two, girl's, printed cotton circle skirts, labeled Fruit of the Loom. $15-20

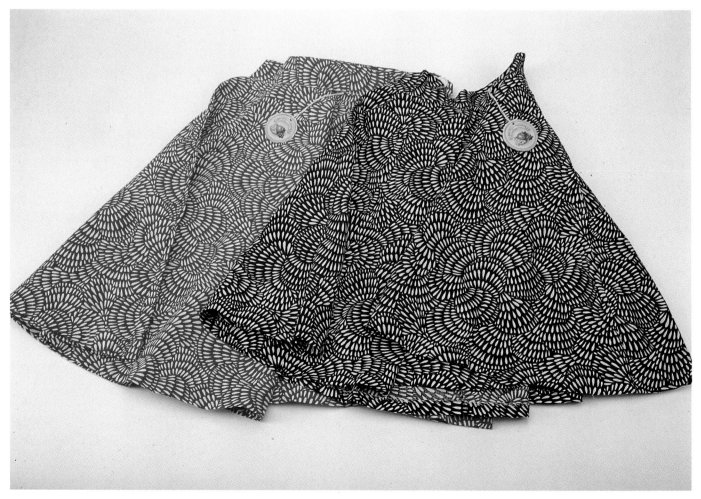

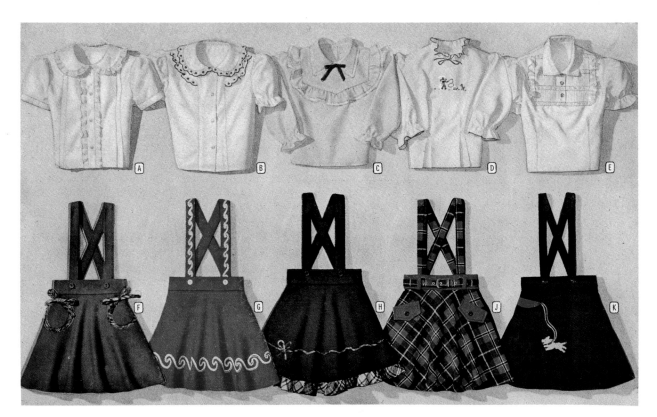

Girls' blouses and skirts with suspenders in solid colors, plaids and novelty patterns fashionable in 1950.

Girl's pleated skirt with suspender straps, made of rayon acetate accented with embroidered decoration, labeled Mandorf Togs, Inc., New York, N.Y. $10-15

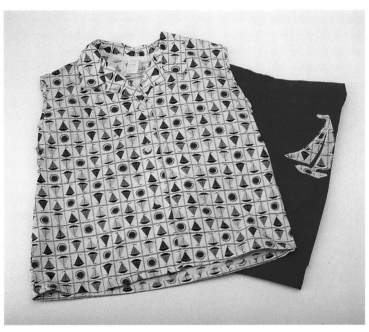

Two-piece summer shorts outfit made of cotton with solid color shorts and printed top, labeled Fruit of the Loom. $8-12 set

Two identical outfits made of cotton with solid color shorts trimmed with striped cuffs, and striped blouses accented with solid color collars, labeled Pert n' Perky. $12-18 set

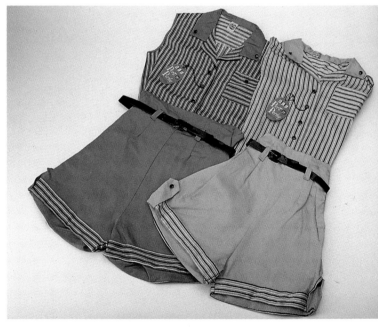

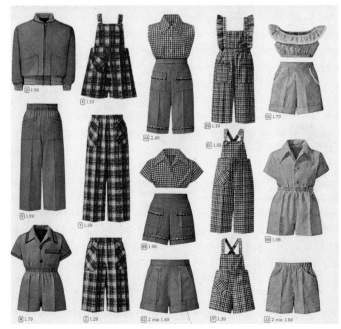

Play clothes made of denim and seersucker styled for boys and girls in 1953.

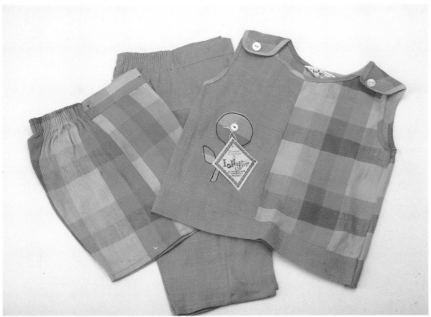

Three-piece summer outfit consisting of shorts, pedal pushers, and sleeveless top made of cotton and rayon, labeled Lolly Togs. $15-20 set

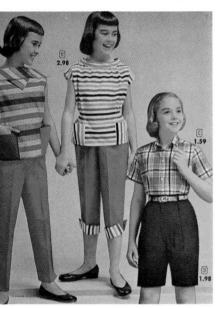

Play clothes made of "easy-care" cottons in solid colors, stripes and plaids designed for 1957.

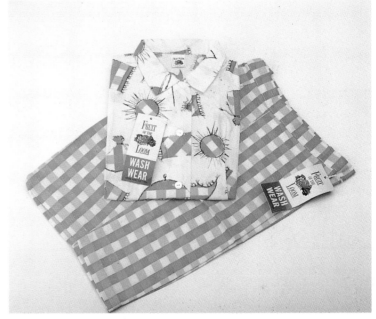

Brightly colored summer shorts outfit made of printed cotton. The set includes a sleeveless blouse and checked Bermuda shorts, labeled Fruit of the Loom. $10-15 set

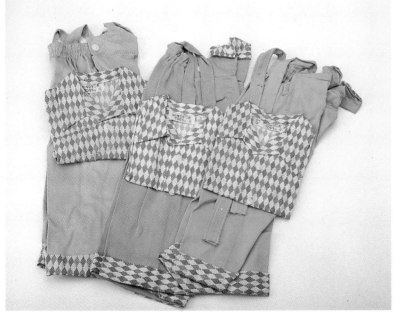

Three, two-piece toddler outfits made of ribbed cotton in different color combinations consisting of overalls and harlequin print tops, labeled Windsor Togs. $15-20 set

73

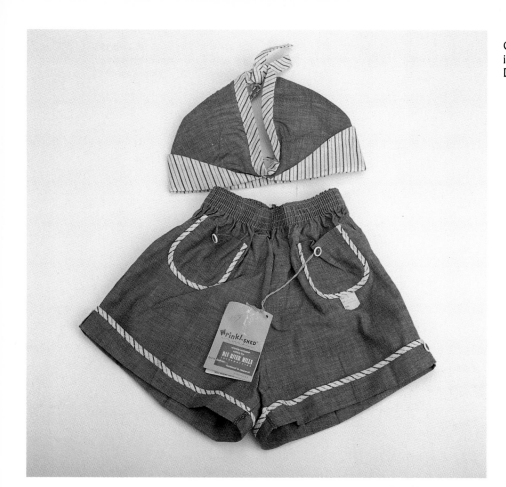

Girl's, two-piece, cotton, play clothes including shorts and a halter top, labeled Dan River. $8-12 set

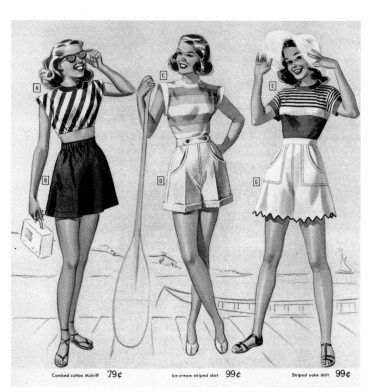

Combed cotton Midriff 79¢   Ice-cream striped shirt 99¢   Striped yoke shirt 99¢

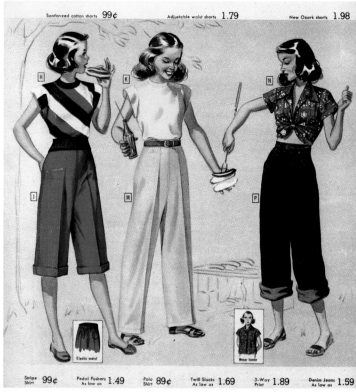

Sanforized cotton shorts 99¢   Adjustable waist shorts 1.79   New Ozark shorts 1.98

Elastic waist

Wear loose

Stripe Shirt 99¢   Pedal Pushers As low as 1.49   Polo Shirt 89¢   Twill Slacks As low as 1.69   3-Way Print 1.89   Denim Jeans As low as 1.59

Sporty "sun and fun" clothes popular for young girls and teens in 1950.

Checks and plaids were used to create these two-piece outfits made of cotton and rayon. This fabric, sometimes termed "sport denim," was extremely popular in the 1950s. $8-12 each

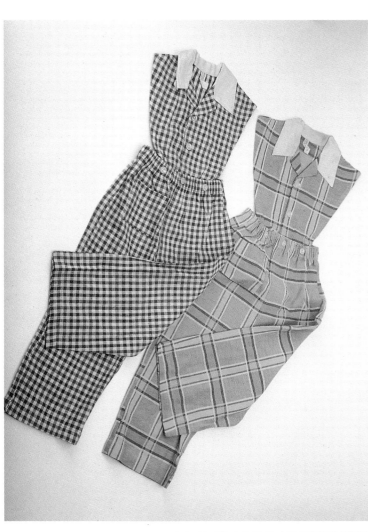

Two, combed cotton knit, pullover tops with silk screened floral design. $10-15 each

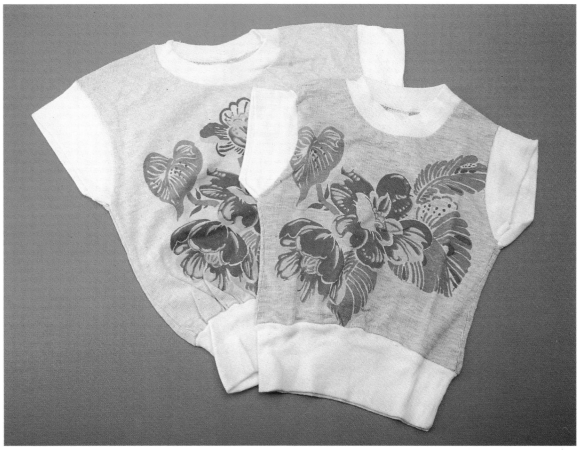

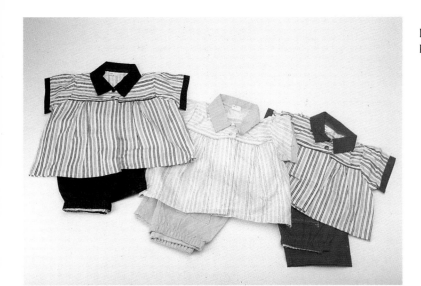

Identical outfits in assorted colors designed with solid color pants and striped smock tops, no label. $12-15 set

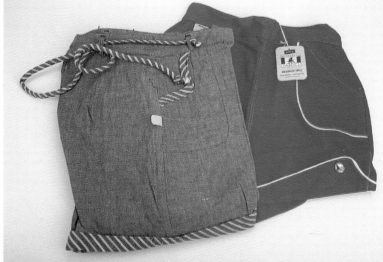

Two pair of lady's summer shorts of Sanforized cotton by Pepperell Fabrics. $10-15 each

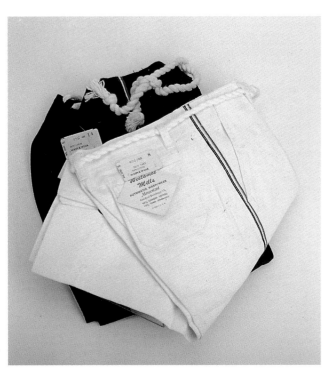

Two pair of girl's, cotton and acrylic, deck pants by Weetamoe Mills. $10-15 each

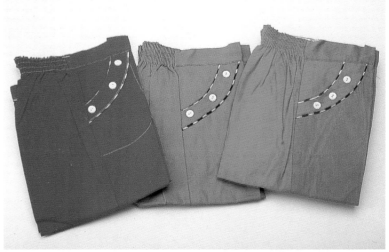

Three pair of solid color cotton pedal pushers accented with striped edging and decorative buttons, labeled Ulster Jr. Rodeo. $8-12 each

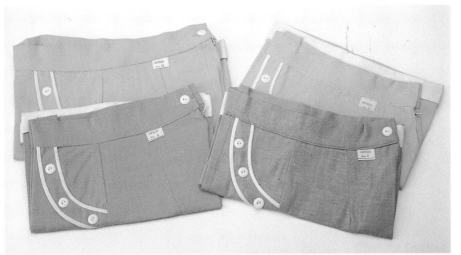

Four pair of shorts made of sport denim in bright colors with white waffled cotton trim. $6-10 each

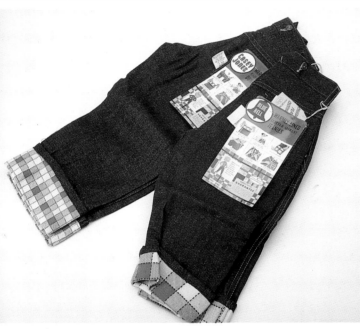

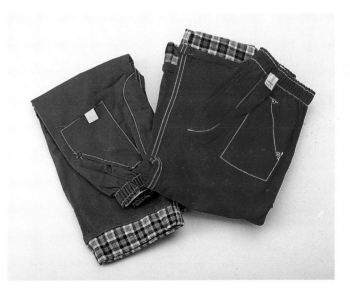

Two pair of warmly lined kiddie's dungarees made of 7 1/4 oz. denim, labeled Casey Jones and Blue Bell. $25-35 each

Western style red and blue cotton pants with plaid flannel lining, decorative stitching, and copper rivets. $15-20 each

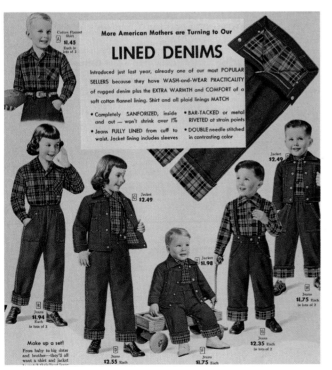

Flannel-lined denim play clothes for children were extremely popular in the 1950s. This assortment, which was designed for both girls and boys, dates from 1953.

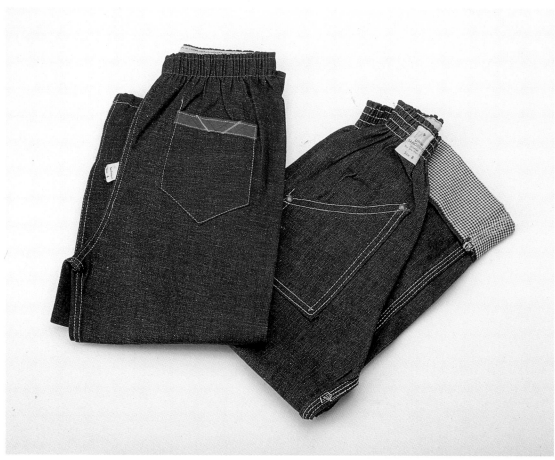

Two pair of girls' light weight denim pants with elastic waist bands and cotton trimmed cuffs and pockets. $20-25 each

This assortment of sportswear designed for the "Young Miss" was fashionable in 1950.

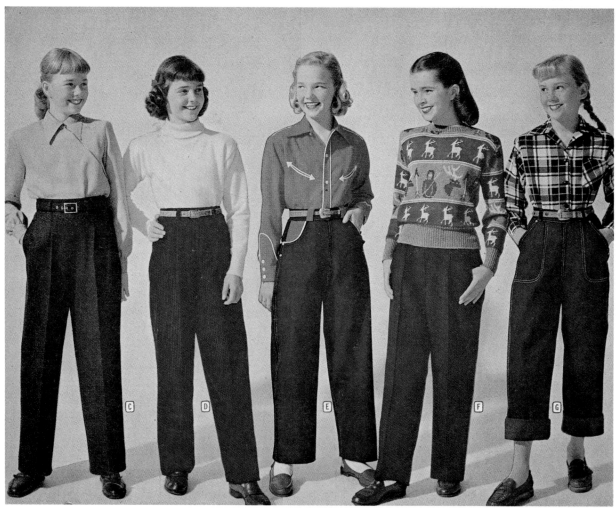

Snug fit, shorty dungarees with decorative
cowboy buttons on the legs. The tag reads:
Dig those crazy Jeans by Salley. $25-35 each

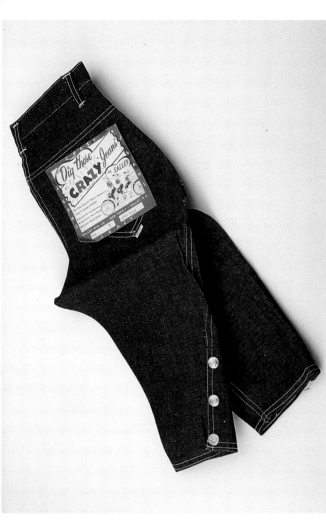

Girl's, pre-shrunk denim jeans with side zipper and
front and back pockets, labeled The H. D. Lee Co.
$35-45

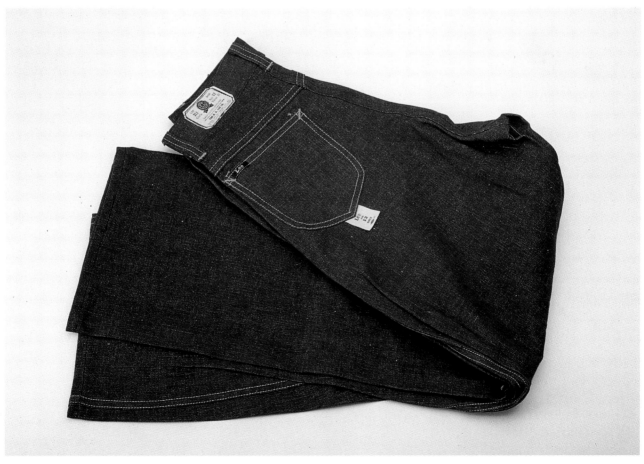

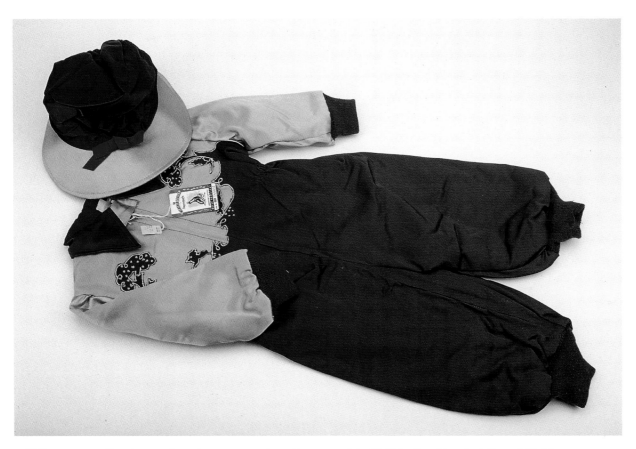

Girl's, water repellent burgundy and grey snow suit and hat, copyright 1943 by Sun Chemical Corp. $45-60

Girls' water-resistant snowsuits in assorted colors and styles popular in 1950.

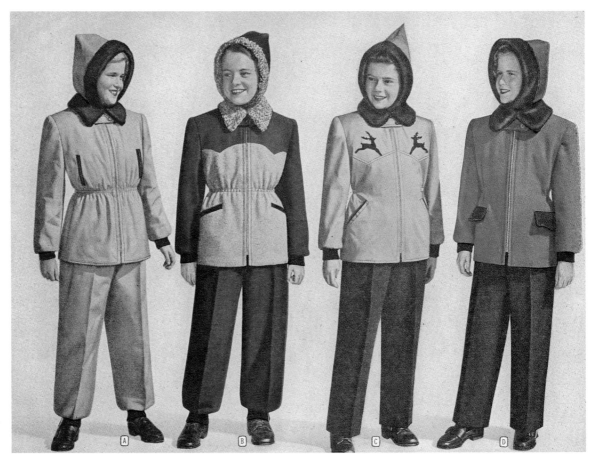

Night Clothes

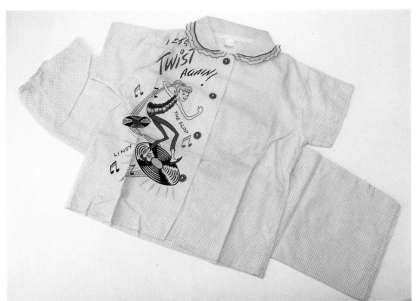

Cotton polka dot pajamas with hand-printed rock & roll motif, no label. $15-20

Red flannel ski pajamas decorated with skiers and skaters, labeled Riegel Flannelette. $7-10

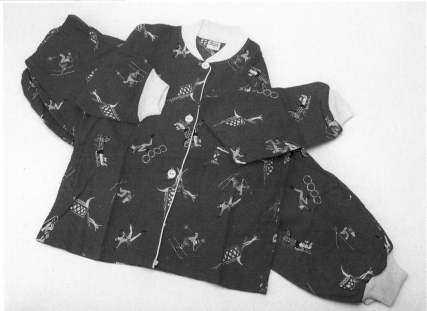

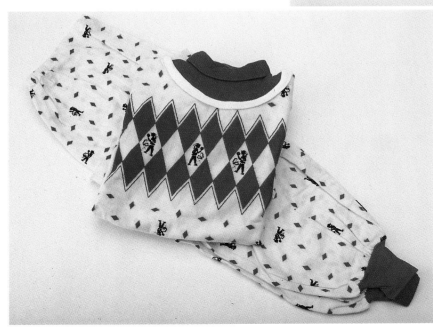

Red and white cotton flannel ski pajamas with diamond pattern, labeled Nite Kraft. $7-10

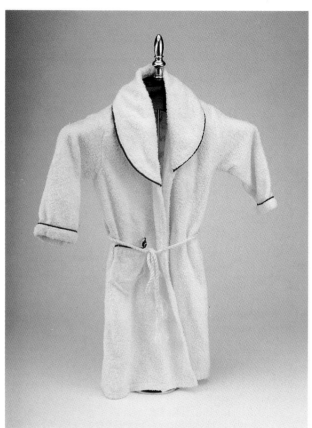

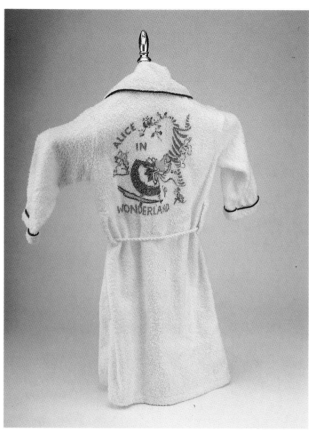

Child's white terry cloth bathrobe with blue piping and stenciled Alice in Wonderland characters on the back. $25-35

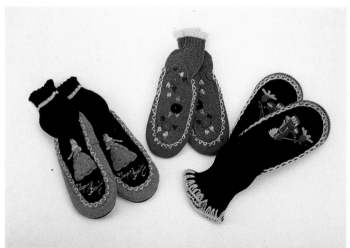

Three pair of children's, wool knit, slipper-socks with embroidered and appliqued decorations. $5-10 pair

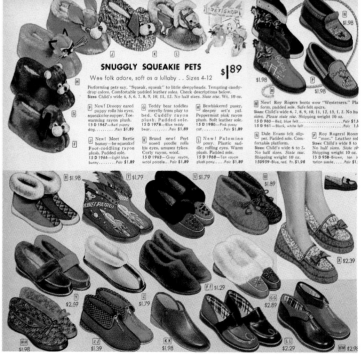

Colorful and whimsical assortment of children's bedroom slippers popular in 1953.

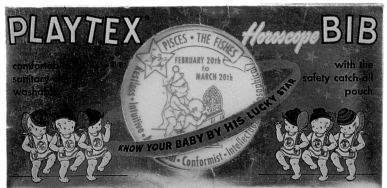

Horoscope bib for baby by Playtex with its original packaging. $7-10

Two, girl's, knit caps with plush trim and chin ties. $4-8 each

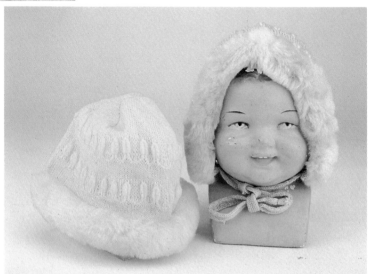

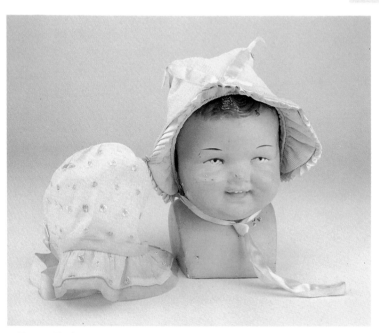

Two, girl's, bonnet-style caps with chin ties, labeled Bonny Babe. $4-8 each

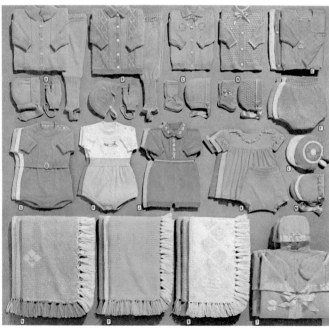

Baby and toddler knitwear, buntings and shawls offered for sale from Montgomery Ward in 1950.

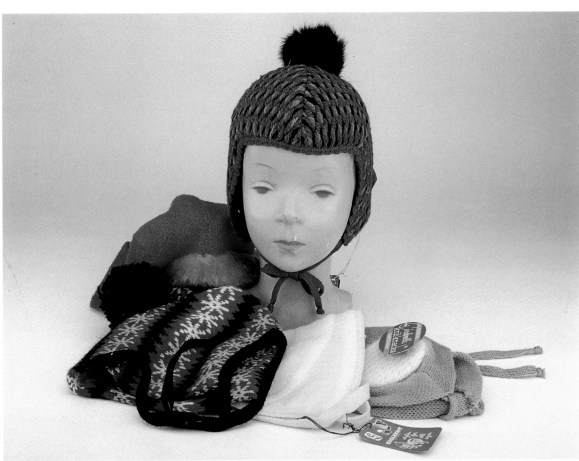

Five, girl's, knit caps with chin ties, labeled Eagleknit and Cinderella knit-knacks Original. $4-8 each

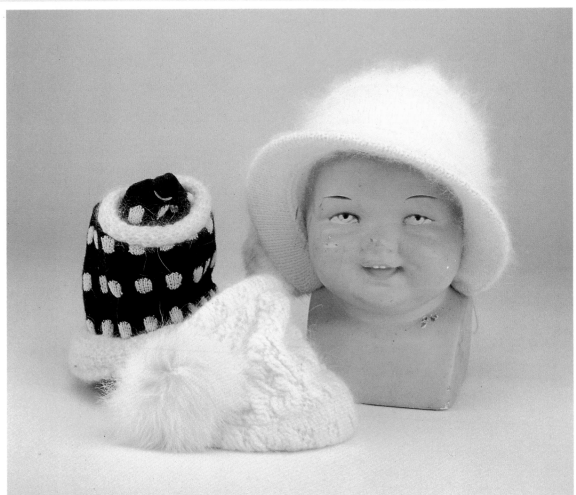

Three girl's, knit caps with chin ties, two made of angora, the other of wool, labeled Cinderella knit-knacks Original. $8-12 each

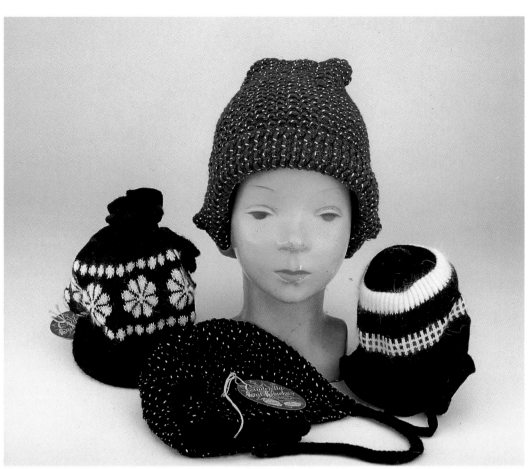

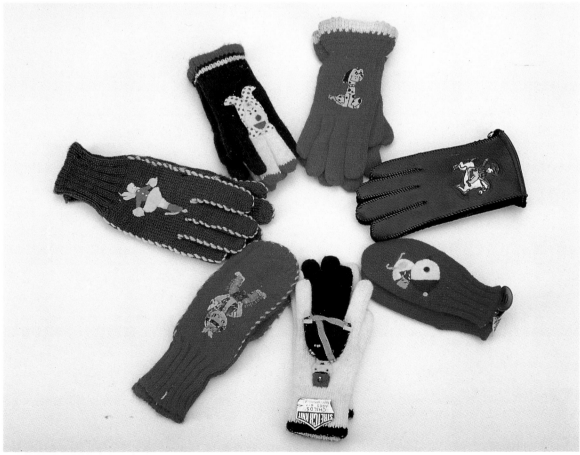

Seven pair of children's gloves with embroidered and appliqued decorations. Six are made of wool knit and one pair of leather-like plastic. $4-8 pair

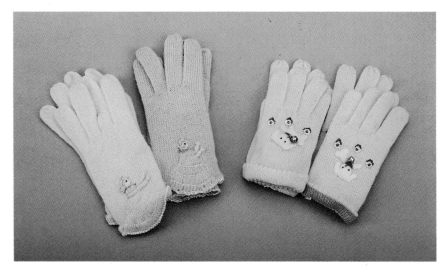

Four pair of little girl's, wool, knit gloves in pastel tones with appliqued decorations. $5-10 pair

Six, white, cotton, child's handkerchiefs printed with the days of the week (excluding Sunday) and a different circus animal on each. They are mounted together on a paper card with printed and movable animals in a circus ring scene. $30-35 set

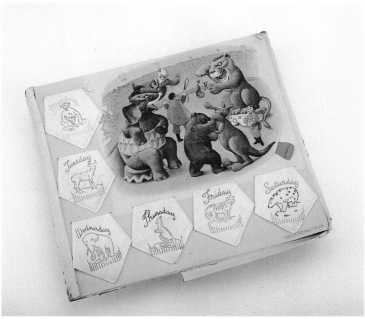

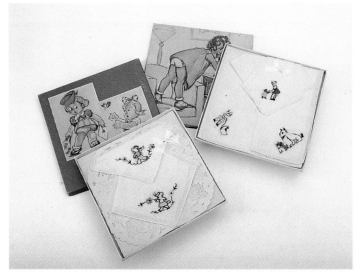

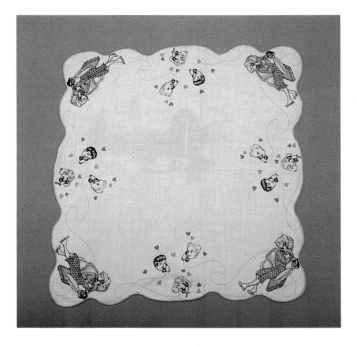

Two sets of young girl's handkerchiefs of white cotton and embroidery, packaged in attractive paper boxes with printed lids. $6-12 each set

White, cotton, handkerchief printed with teenagers talking on the telephone and edged with pink embroidery thread. $3-5

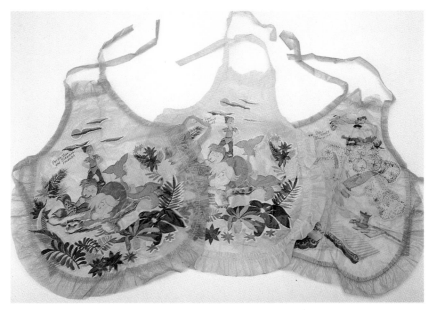

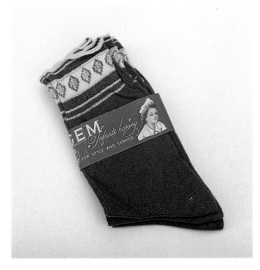

Girl's colored cotton socks with patterned cuffs, labeled Gem Hosiery. $1-3 each pair

Three child's aprons in pink and yellow, plastic decorated with Peter Pan, Tinker Bell, and friends, marked Walt Disney Productions. $20-25 each

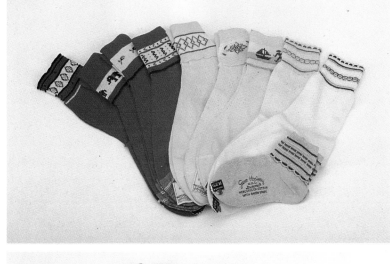

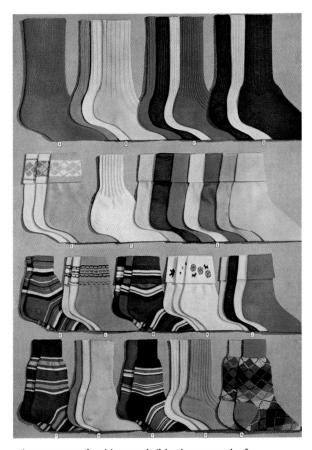

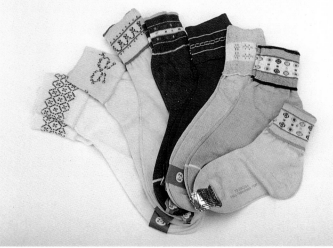

Assortment of anklets and ribbed crew socks for children in solid colors, blazer stripes and sporty argyles from 1950.

Assorted girl's cotton socks with patterned cuffs labeled Durene by Sturdywear Hose, Belnord Sox, and Gem Hosiery. $1-3 each pair.

Shoes

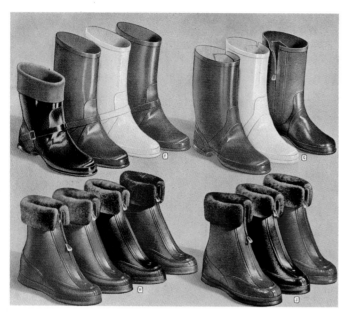

Rubber footwear for children in assorted colors and styles offered for sale in 1950.

These leather shoes designed for children in 1953 look almost identical to those designed today.

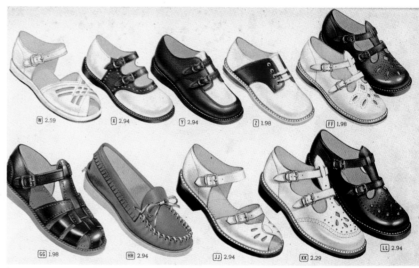

W 2.59   X 2.94   Y 2.94   Z 1.98   FF 1.98

GG 1.98   HH 2.94   JJ 2.94   KK 2.29   LL 2.94

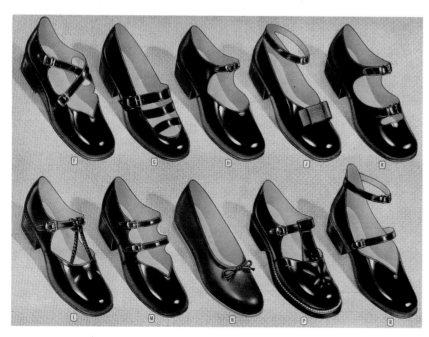

Dress shoes for girls made of smooth and patent leather offered for sale in 1950.

Lingerie

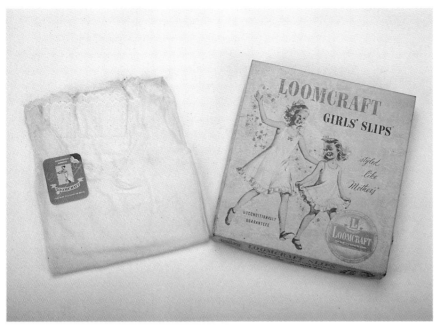

White cotton slips for little girls with cotton eyelet decoration defining the neckline and the hemline. Labeled: Loomcraft "styled like mother's," in their original box. $3-6 each

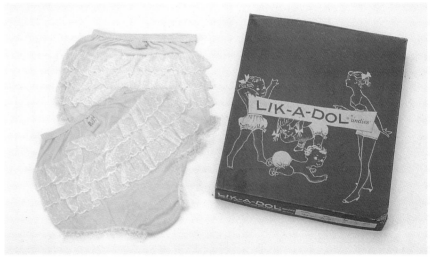

Little girl's underpants made of acetate with nylon lace trim, labeled Lik-A-Dol. Presented with its original box. $1-3 per pair

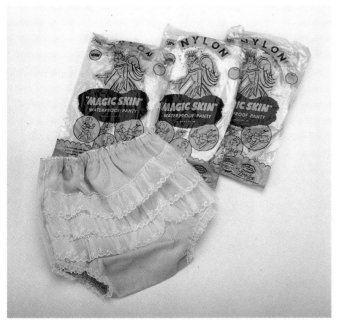

"Magic Skin" waterproof panty made of 100% nylon and rubber lined in green, yellow, blue & white, labeled Styled by Birdy Products. $1-3 per pair

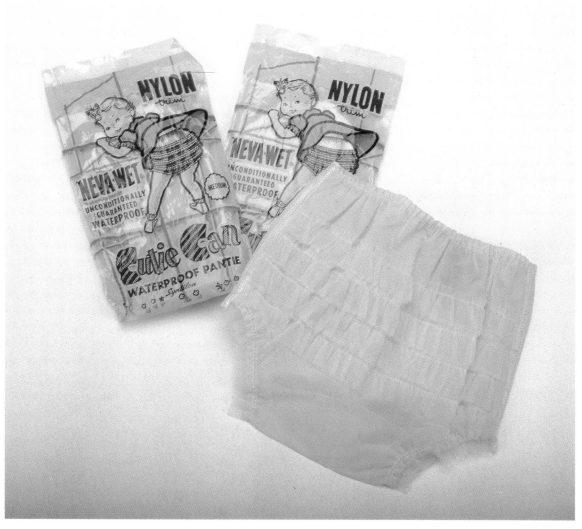

"Cutie Can" waterproof panties for babies in pink and yellow with nylon trim, labeled "Neva-Wet" Waterproof Pantie Styled by Pageant Und. Co. $1-3 per pair

Assortment of waterproof pants for babies, all made by Playtex and still in their original packaging. $2-4 each

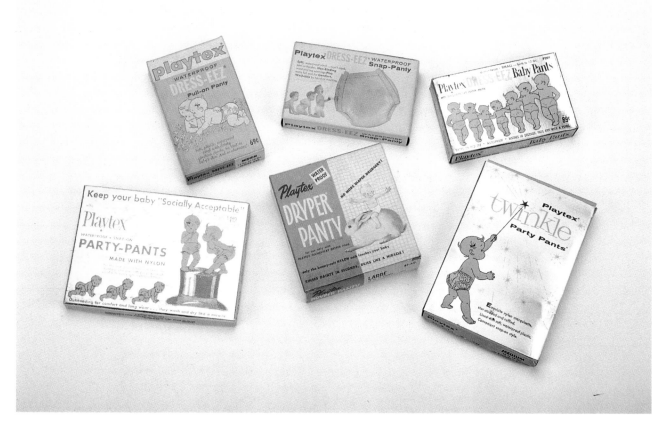

Chapter Three
Fashions For MenShirts

Shirt styles for men in the 1950s was a broad category consisting of many designs utilizing many different fabrics. The basic dress shirt was made of cotton broadcloth or oxford cloth. Later in the decade, DuPont Dacron and Egyptian cotton were used. The colors were usually the basic white, light blue, light pink, pale yellow, light beige or tan. Solid colors were always popular in addition to neat thin stripes, small checks, pin dots or small all-over prints. In 1955, dress shirts became a little more elaborate and pleated fronts with French cuffs entered the fashion scene.

While the body of the shirt remained pretty standard, vast differences were found on the collar designs. In the early-to-mid 1950s, medium and long point collars were fashionable as well as short to medium widespread collars. Button-down collars, especially on oxford shirts were common. Collars for the button-down variety were either pointed or rounded. Rounded collars were either secured to the shirt with buttons or they were designed with eyelets and secured with a collar pin.

In the 1950s, sportswear became big business. Even though the sportswear category was the "youngest category in the apparel industry", by 1956 it became the leader in promotion and fashion development. So much variety was found in men's sportswear in this decade largely due to the fact that consumers were aware of being "leisure conscious" at this time. Many original ideas came from California and many American designers got their inspiration from the Italian designers.

In the early 1950s, lustrous rayon gabardine was hot. Sport shirts were designed with two-way medium to long point sport collars to be worn either open or closed. Double front pockets were almost always part of the shirt design and they were either flap pockets or button-down patch pockets. Long sleeve and short sleeve variations were offered for all seasons. Colors like maroon, navy, gray, light blue, light green, gold, spice brown and forest green were common. Salmon and pink were added to the color spectrum and these colors became extremely fashionable around 1955.

Two-toned color combinations were ultra stylish. Some designs included the body of the shirt one color, and the collar, cuffs and pocket flaps another color. Popular color combinations included gray and maroon, pink and black, or purple and gray.

Spiegel offered some unusual sport shirts in 1950 made of gabardine. These designs included button shield fronts, jacket-style shirts with elastic waistbands, two-toned angle-zip shirts and diagonal zipper front shirts. In the same year, the National Bellas Hess Company offered through their mail-order catalog washable gabardine shirts with laced bib fronts, round spread collars and knit waistbands designed for a "snug fit". Color combinations like pink and black or purple and gray were featured. Gabardine shirts were also offered in plaids, large checks or splash checks.

Besides gabardine, sport shirts of the 1950s were also made of cotton and silk blends, cotton and rayon blends, printed madras cloth, acetate, cotton crinkle crepe, nubby cotton poplin, cool cotton mesh, Orlon and rayon blends and cotton and wool flannel, to name a few.

In 1956, shirts made of cotton and acetate, and silks and iridescent yarns created unique and lustrous new looks. In the same year, *Apparel Arts* stated that:

> Knitwear reflects new continental ideas in styling. Shawl collars are news in sweaters along with dickey or bib fronts. The shirt sweater is expected to attain great favor in Orlon but crew neck pullovers are still number one in demand in long-sleeve and sleeveless styles. Coat sweaters in coarse weaves will also become a style factor. The low-cut sweater vest is gaining ground.

Unusual sport shirts also spawned unusual collars. Names like Italian collar, continental collar, gaucho collar, curved collar and blunt point collar were stylish.

By 1955, manufacturers and designers looking for novel shirt ideas became focused on the collar style, the fabric pattern and color to create the perfect look to stimulate consumer interest. Pink was still a hot color for men's shirts, but other colors like pale blue, mint green and coral were gaining popularity. As jacket lapels were beginning to slim down, the size of the shirt collar followed suit. Patterned fabrics were becoming more common especially checks and stripes in unusual color combinations.

The designer craze of the 1950s found its way into men's sportswear. In 1957, designer original sport shirts by Marlboro included what their ad describes as..."a masterpiece of muted elegance...Panel-Rama...the pattern that parallels a pure satin center with narrower stripes of satin". A year earlier, fashion news in men's sport shirts for the summer of 1956 was panel stripes. When the wide stripe ran horizontal, the effect was a broader look; when the panel was vertical, a taller look was achieved. A year later, satin was tastefully used and labeled a designer original. Panel stripes allowed the designer to use his creativity.

Marlboro Shirt Company also advertised shirts designed by Tammis Keefe, a famed artist of the period. Her unique collection included shirts with small prints depicting Nordic shields, helmets, coins and crown jewels.

In the summer of 1951, tribal prints, inspired by the "Dark Continent" of Africa were showing up on men's sportswear and beachwear. Tropical prints from island paradises like Hawaii and the Caribbean were gaining excitement in the fashion industry. Sport shirts, swim shorts and matched sport sets were highly fashionable and almost always made of rayon, occasionally made of cotton. By the late 1950s, native prints inspired from the West Indies were featured on sport shirts and beachwear. Batik and screen prints were extremely stylish.

Western shirts for men were also popular in the 1950s. Authentic styling with two-toned color combinations, colorful embroidery and piped trim were highly fashionable. The shirts were occasionally styled with snap buttons or ocean pearl shank buttons and tapered cuffs. The cuffs varied from three snaps to what was called a five-snap Caballero cuff. The pocket styles also varied to include dart, flap, saddle bag or two-point Arizona wing pockets.

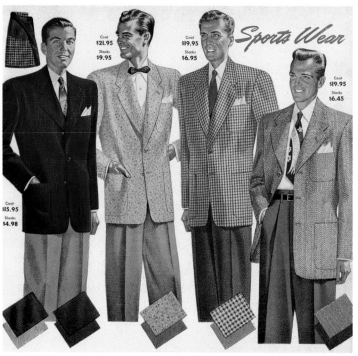

Tailored "Sports Wear" for men in corduroy, tweed, check and herringbone popular in 1951.

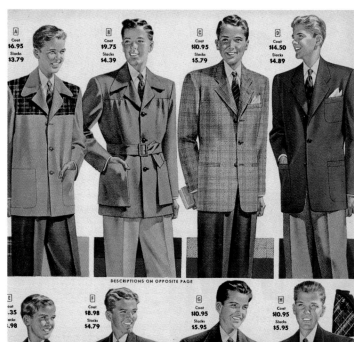

Leisure jackets and sport coats offered for young men in 1951 made of corduroy in solid colors and two-toned color combinations.

92

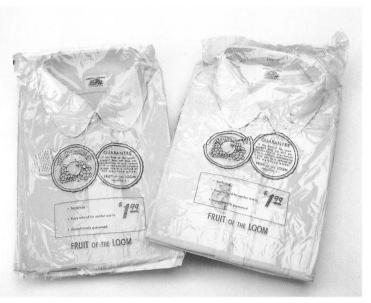

Two cotton shirts in their original packaging, made with rounded, button down collars, labeled Fruit of the Loom. $20-25 each

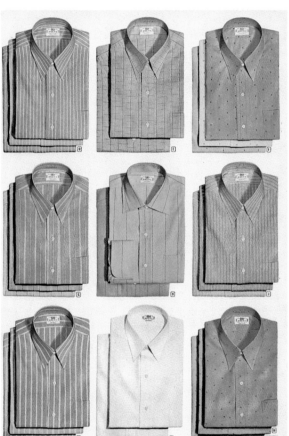

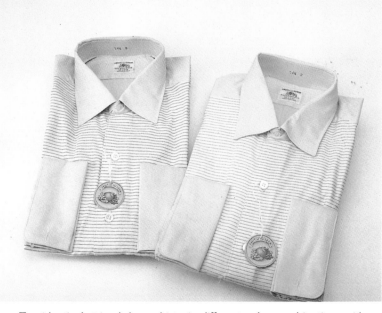

Two identical striped dress shirts, in different color combinations with solid color collar and cuffs, labeled Fruit of the Loom. $30-35 each

Cotton dress shirts in solid colors and assorted stripes with regular and spread collars styled for 1950 and sold through Montgomery Ward.

Long sleeve broadcloth dress shirts and ties offered for sale from Spiegel in 1950.

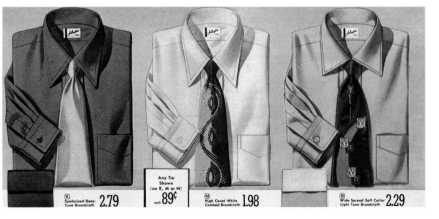

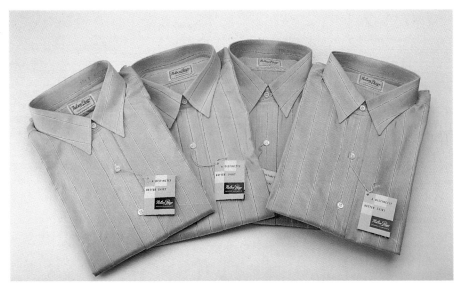

Four sanforized cotton dress shirts with vertical stripes, in different color combinations, labeled Nelson Paige. $25-35 each

Trio of men's shirts with classic 1950s tailoring, made of rayon and acetate, labeled Fruit of the Loom. $85-100 each

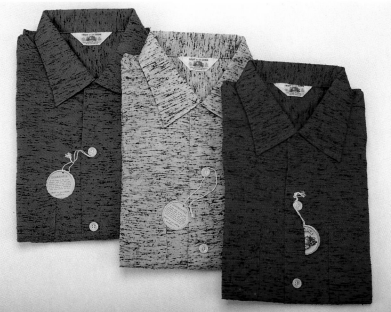

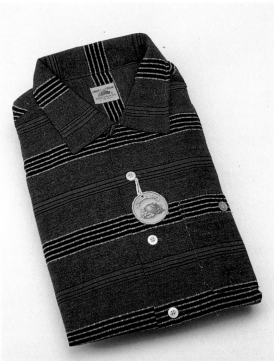

Four-toned, long sleeve rayon sport shirt with horizontal striping, labeled Fruit of the Loom. $45-75

Four-toned, long sleeve, cotton sport shirt, with horizontal striping, labeled Fruit of the Loom. $35-50

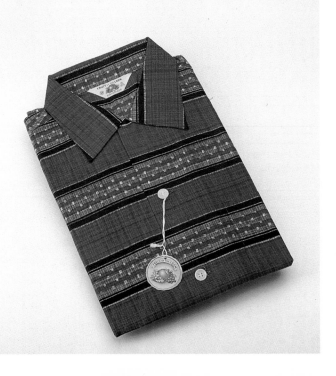

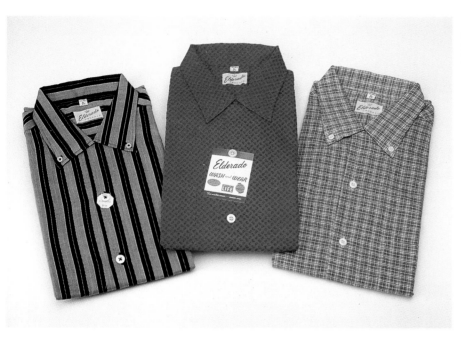

Assortment of men's cotton shirts with plaid, striped, and small paisley prints, labeled Eldorado Casuals. $35-50 each

Cotton sport shirt designed with an Italian collar and black and red vertical stripes, labeled Fruit of the Loom. $35-50

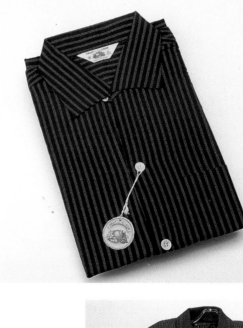

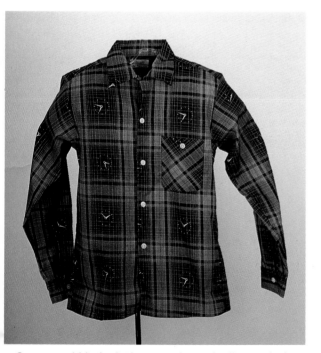

Orange and black plaid cotton shirt with all-over clock motif, labeled Mohawk Sportwear. $35-50

Burgundy and gray knit sport shirt made of rayon and cotton, labeled Wings Knitwear. $30-50

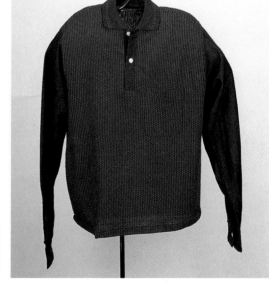

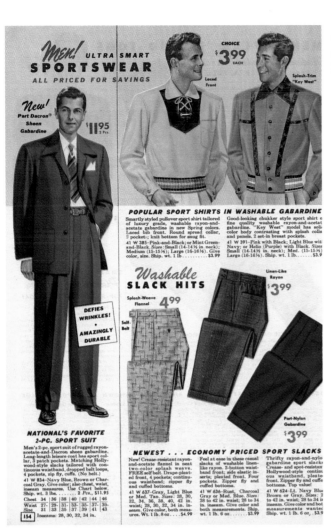

Trend-setting clothing offered for men in the 1955 Spring and Summer National Bellas Hess mail-order catalog.

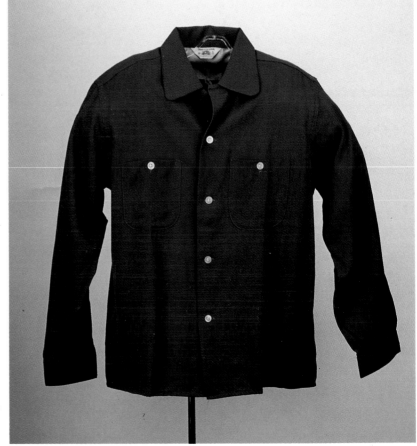

Long sleeve, gray rayon gabardine sport shirt with rounded collar and double front pockets, labeled Fruit of the Loom. $65-95

96

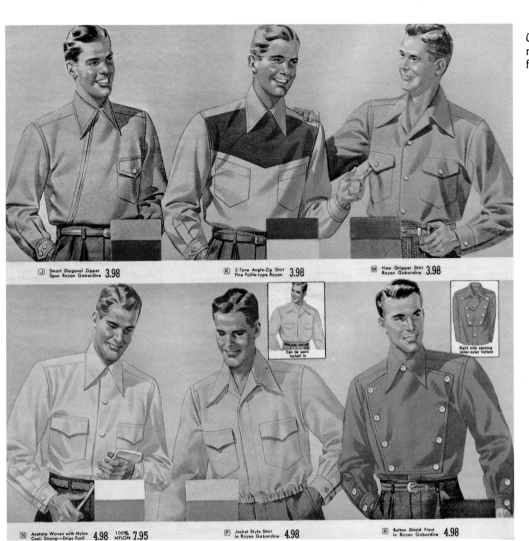

J Smart Diagonal Zipper
Spun Rayon Gabardine 3.98

K 2-Tone Angle-Zip Shirt
Fine Faille-type Rayon 3.98

M New Gripper Shirt
Rayon Gabardine 3.98

Can be worn tucked in

Right side opening inner-outer button

N Acetate Woven with Nylon
Cool, Strong—Dries Fast! 4.98   100%
NYLON 7.95

P Jacket Style Shirt
in Rayon Gabardine 4.98

R Button Shield Front
in Rayon Gabardine 4.98

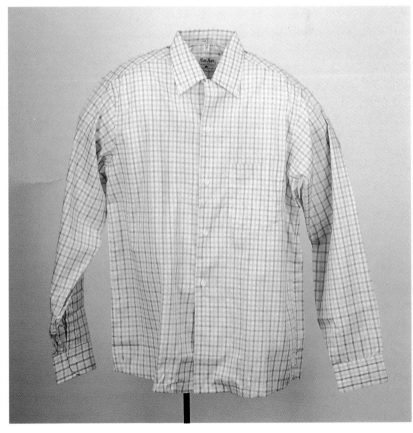

Three-toned, plaid, long-sleeve cotton shirt with button down collar, labeled Mark Twain Exclusive Design. $30-45

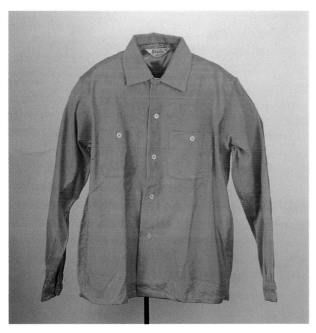

Salmon colored corduroy shirt with double front pockets, labeled Wilshire. $60-95

Two plaid flannel shirts from the early and mid-1950s by Fruit of the Loom and Kenberry. $35-45 each

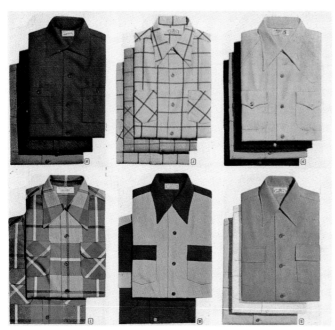

Sport shirts styled for the 1950-1951 Fall and Winter season made of gabardine, slubbed poplin, rayon and cotton chambray.

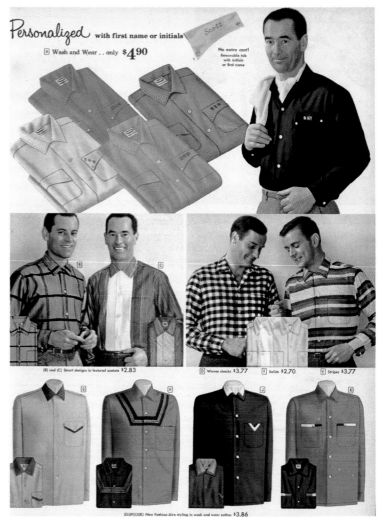

Exceptionally stylish men's long sleeve sport shirts designed for the 1958-1959 Fall and Winter season.

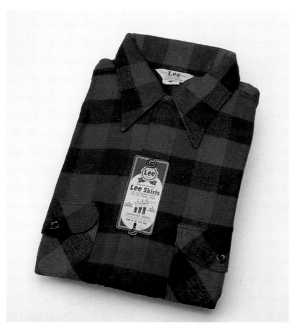

Black and red checked flannel shirt with double button-down flap pockets, labeled Lee Union Made. $35-45

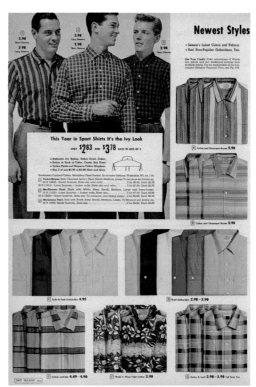

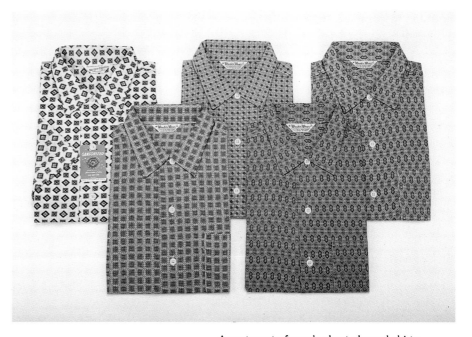

Assortment of men's short-sleeved shirts made of Sanforized cotton with interesting geometric prints, labeled Designer Collection. $ 25-35 each

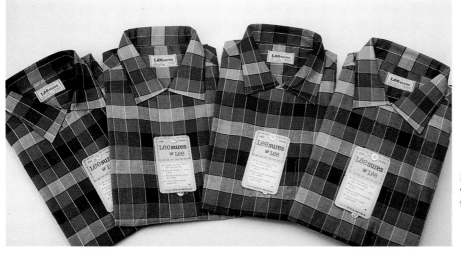

Four identical long sleeve, cotton sport shirts with plaid designs in different color combinations, labeled Leesures by Lee. $35-50 each

Three acetate, checked sport shirts in different color combinations, labeled Fruit of the Loom. $30-40 each

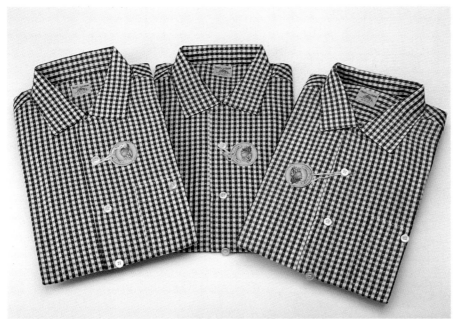

Two long-sleeve, two-toned checked shirts, with wide spread collars and double-flap front pockets, labeled Lion of Troy. $35-45 each

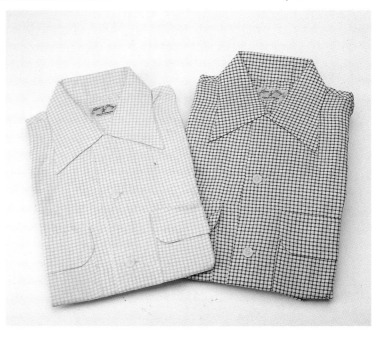

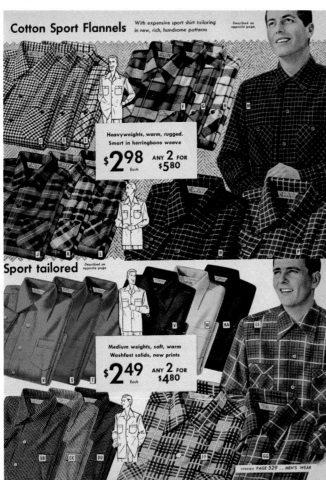

Cotton Sport Flannels With expensive sport shirt tailoring in new, rich, handsome patterns

Described on opposite page.

Heavyweights, warm, rugged. Smart in herringbone weave

$**2**⁹⁸ Each ANY **2** FOR $⁵80

Sport tailored Described on opposite page.

Medium weights, soft, warm Washfast solids, new prints

$**2**⁴⁹ Each ANY **2** FOR $⁴80

OPENING PAGE 529 .. MEN'S WEAR

"Pilgrim" brand medium and heavyweight flannel shirts in plaids, checks and solid colors offered from Sears in 1953.

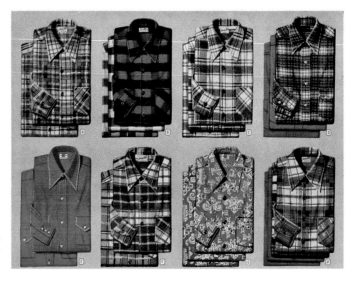

Wool and cotton flannel shirts in solid colors, plaids, checks and prints popular in 1950.

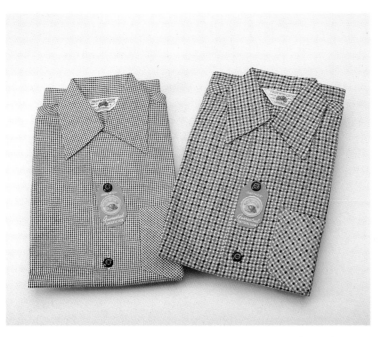

Two long sleeve checked shirts made of cotton, labeled Fruit of the Loom. $40-50 each

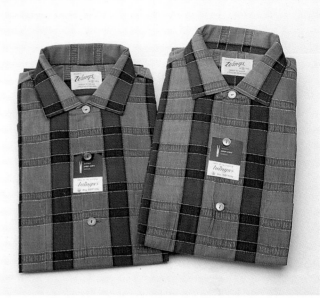

Two cotton shirts with plaid designs in different color combinations, accented with ornamental stitching, labeled Silver Wings. $35-45 each

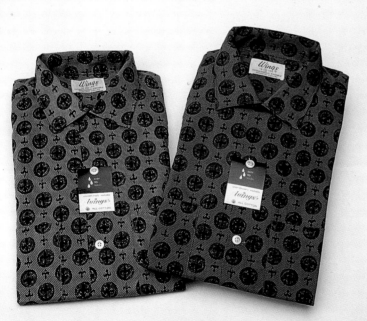

Two cotton sport shirts with fleur-de-lis patterns in different color combinations, labeled Wings. Unconditionally washable, with wingstay collar. $25-35 each

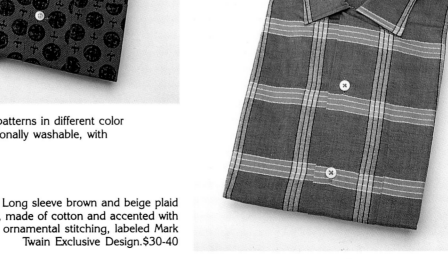

Long sleeve brown and beige plaid shirt, made of cotton and accented with ornamental stitching, labeled Mark Twain Exclusive Design. $30-40

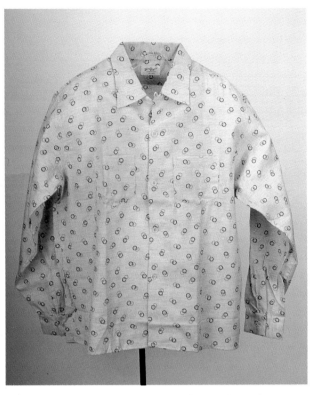

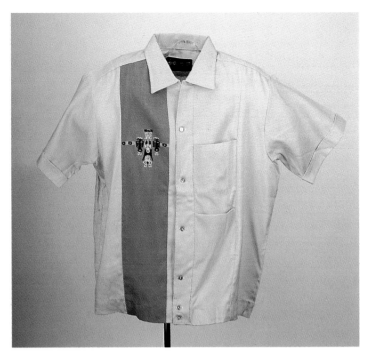

Paneled two-toned sport shirt with Aztec motif, made of rayon, labeled A Nat Nast Creation. $35-45

Interlocking circles decorate this classic 1950s shirt made of a wearever fabric Flannaire - a luxurious blend of 96% cotton and 4% wool, labeled Town Topic. $25-35

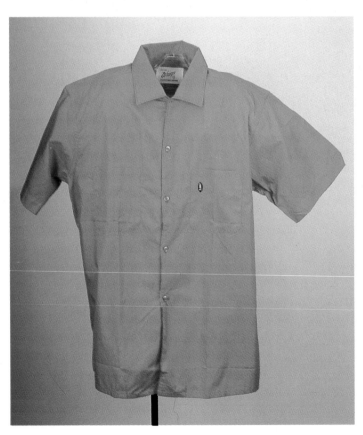

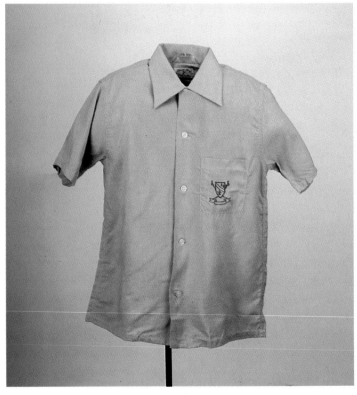

Pale aqua short sleeve sport shirt made of rayon with heraldic embroidery on pocket, labeled Lion of Troy. $30-35

Orange sport shirt made of 100% supima cotton, decorated with embroidery on pocket, labeled Silver Wings. $25-35

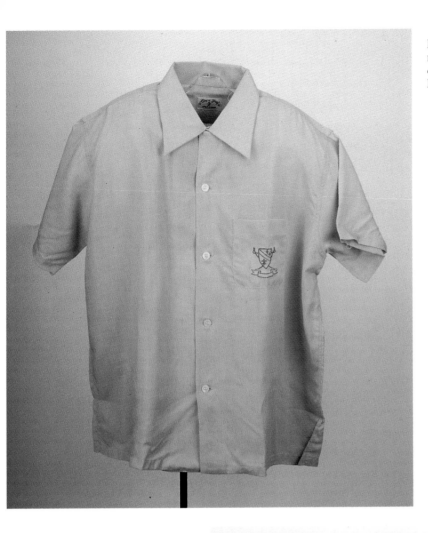

Beige short sleeve sport shirt
made of rayon with heraldic
embroidery on pocket, labeled
Lion of Troy. $30-35

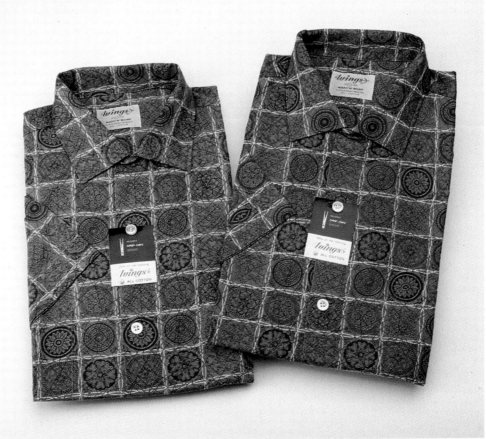

Two abstract printed cotton
short sleeve shirts with
spread collars, labeled
Wings. $30-35 each

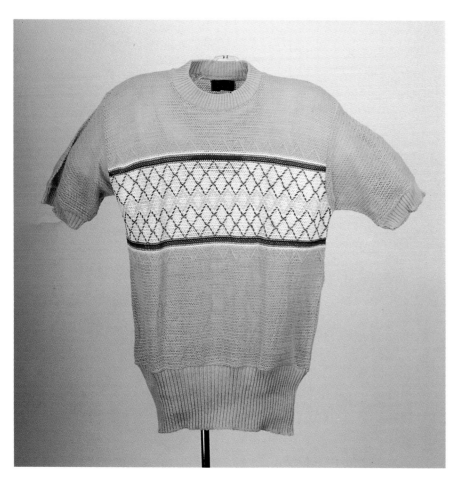

Beige cotton cable knit pullover with horizontal zig-zag stitching forming diamond patterns, labeled Allen-A Sportwear. $35-50

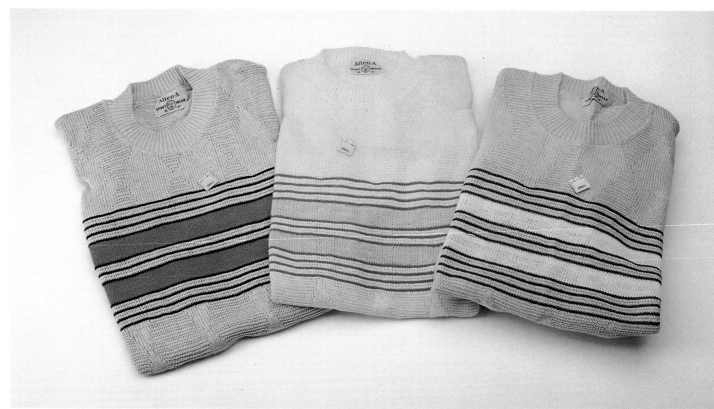

Three men's cable knit pullovers with unusual zig-zag patterns, labeled Allen-A Sportswear. $35-50 each

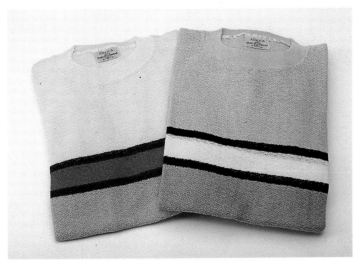

Two cotton knit pullovers with four-toned horizontal striping, labeled Allen-A Sportswear. $35-50 each

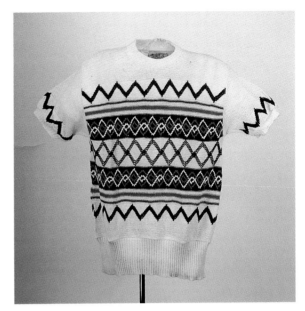

Short sleeve cable knit pullover with red and blue zig-zag embroidery, labeled Delsea Country Club Sport Shirt. $40-50

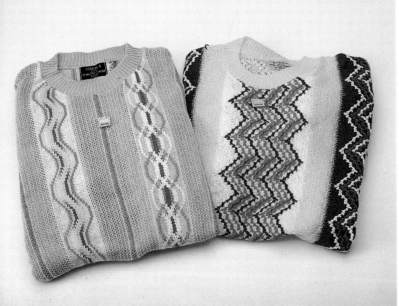

Two cable knit cotton pullover sweaters with bright colored vertical designs, labeled Allen-A Sportswear. $40-50 each

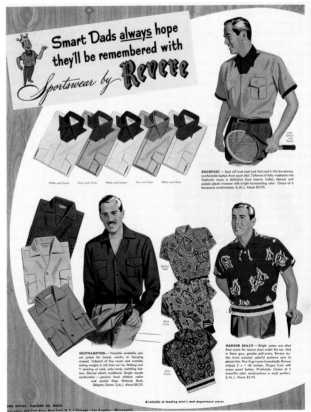

"Revere" sportswear for men advertised in *Esquire*, July, 1951.

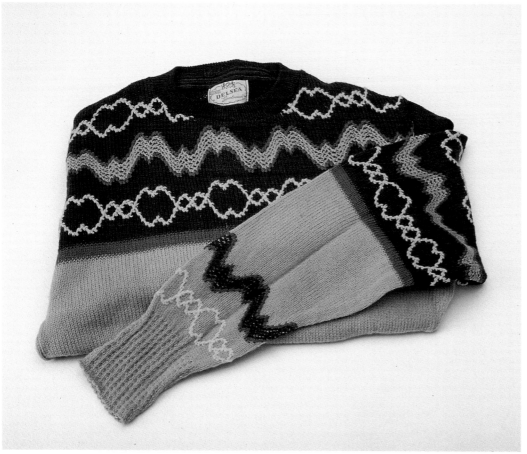

Four-toned wool knit sweater with zig-zag stitching, labeled Delsea Sportswear. $40-50

Two solid color knit shirts made of cotton and decorated with ornamental trim, labeled Glen Hall Sportswear. $25-35

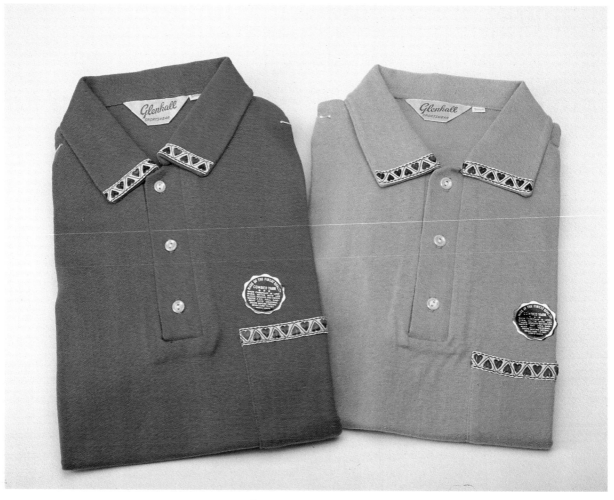

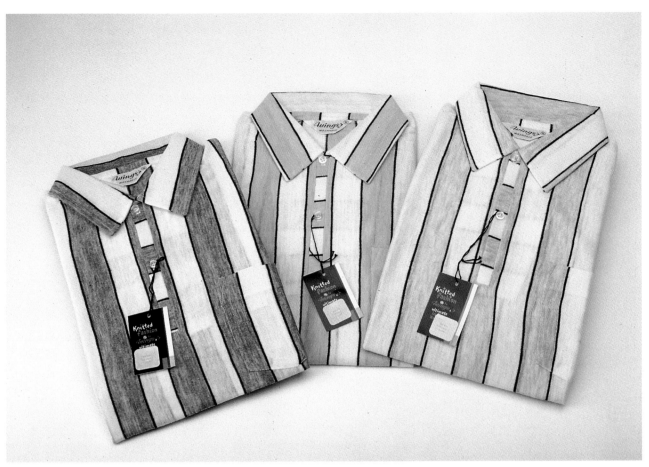

Trio of three-toned knit shirts with vertical
stripes, made of rayon and acrylic fibers, labeled
Wings. $25-30 each

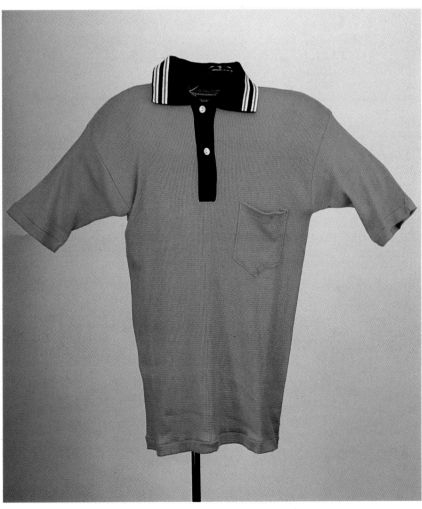

Turquoise knit sport shirt with
red, white and black trim,
labeled Delsea Country Club
Sport Shirt. $30-35

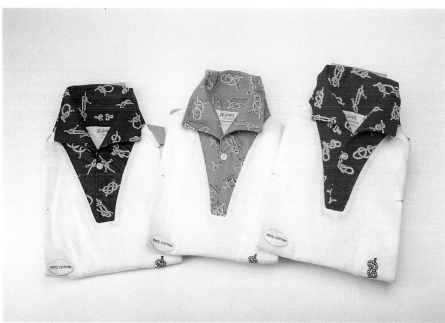

Trio of summer short sleeve knit shirts made of cotton with nautical designs, accented with embroidery, labeled Wings Knitwear. $25-30

Short sleeve black knit sport shirt made of cotton and Rayon with Italian collar and heraldic patch, labeled Glenhall Sportwear. $20-30

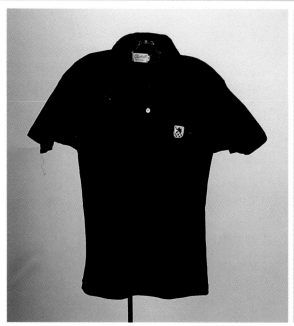

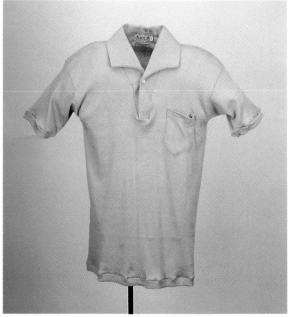

Gray short sleeve sport shirt of combed cotton with Italian collar, labeled Delsea Country Club Sport Shirt. $20-30

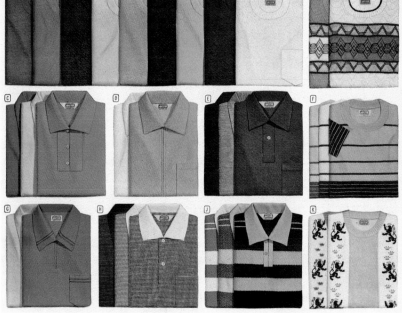

Crew necks, cable knits, zipper fronts and button-down knit shirts in solids, stripes and novelty prints fashionable in 1955.

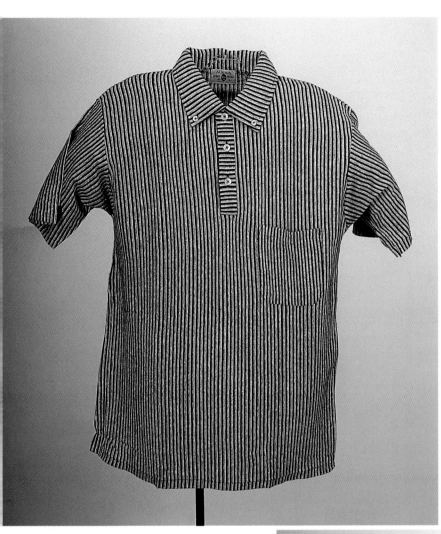

Three-toned knit sport shirt with button down collar, labeled Allen-A Sportswear. $20-30

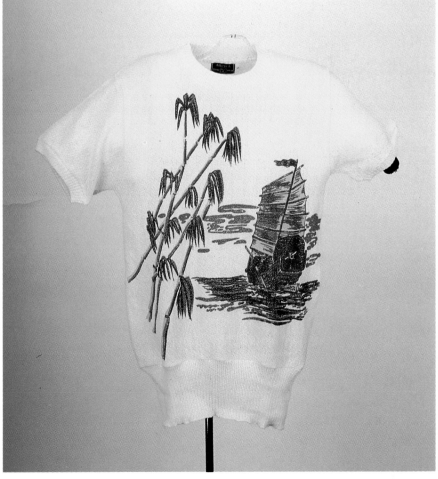

Bright yellow cotton pullover with hand screened oriental scene, labeled by Allen-A Sportwear. $45-55

win one of 25 thrilling all-expense-paid vacations

to the romantic Caribbean

...or 326 **valuable cash prizes!**

go
*Carribean**
with
Catalina

Imagine winning an all-expense-paid vacation trip to the Caribbean wonderland—inspiration for Catalina's new, spirited Carribean Collection! Beautiful new designs, gay sun-filled colors, fanciful patterns and fabrics, all created with a true Caribbean flavor!*

It's fun! It's easy to enter!

Ask for contest blank in the swimwear department of leading department stores and men's shops in your city.

Shown above: *SEA KELP, California hand-print Sandskin Cabana set. Trunk features Catalina's exclusive patented 3-in-1 Lastex pouch, knitted support. From Catalina's exciting new Carribean* Collection.*

You'll fly via luxurious Pan American World Airways —stay at the finest hotels!

LOOK FOR THE **FLYING FISH**

Catalina, Inc., from Los Angeles, California sponsored a contest in 1951 for a free Caribbean vacation. The Caribbean was the company's inspiration for its new sportswear and beachwear line.

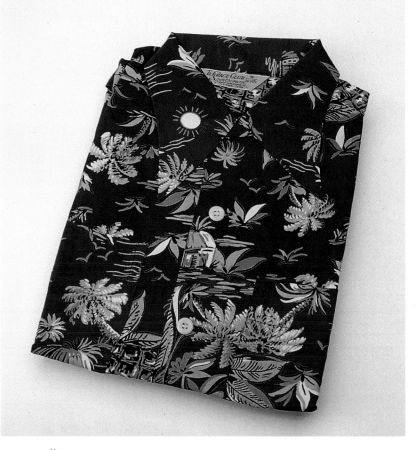

Hawaiian style pineapple print shirt made of rayon, labeled Terrace Club Sportswear. $85-125

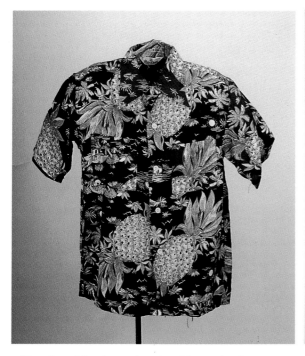

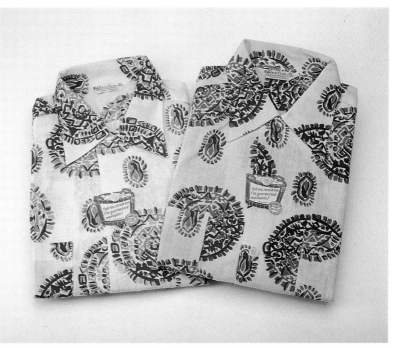

Hawaiian-style pineapple print shirt made of rayon, labeled Beau Crest Handwashable. $85-125

Two rayon sport shirts with tribal prints in different color combinations, labeled Terrace Club Sportswear. $40-50 each

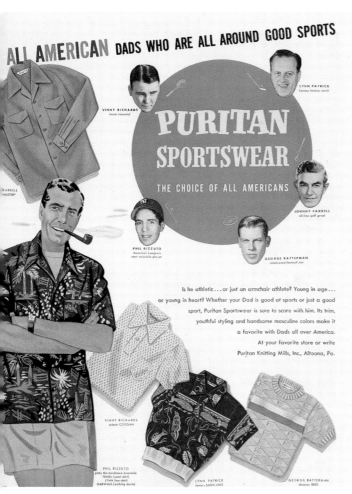

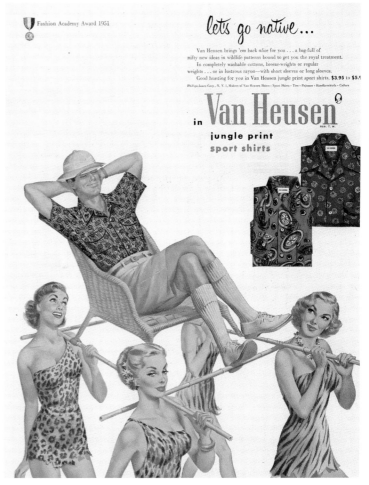

Sportswear by "Puritan" advertised in *Esquire*, July, 1951. Famous athletes were used in this ad as a merchandising technique to sell the clothes.

Sport shirts by "Van Heusen" in exotic jungle prints as advertised in *Esquire* in July of 1951.

Western wear was extremely stylish in the
1950s for men, women and children.
These men's shirts could be made at home
with McCall's patterns which were advertised in 1953.

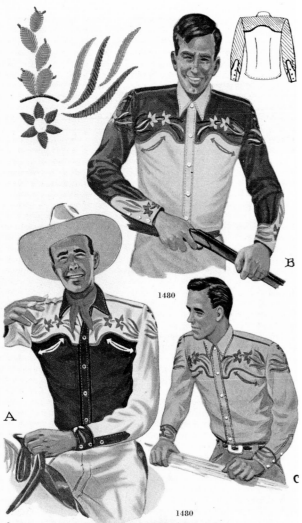

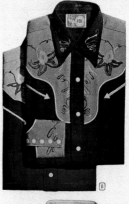

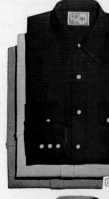

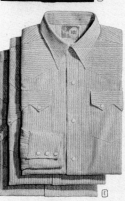

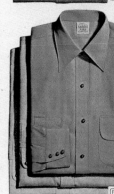

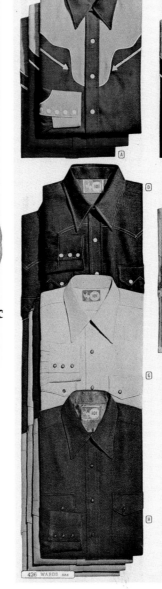

Authentic Western Style Shirts

A RAYON GABARDINE. Made in the West. Striking two-tone Rodeo styling, trimmed with white piping. Has snap buttons, tapered five-button cuffs, dart-slash-pockets, regular collar and full length tails. Colors: Green with Gray, Maroon with Gray, Brown with Tan. Dry clean. Sizes: 14, 14½, 15, 15½, 16, 16½, 17-in. neck. Ship. wt. 1 lb. 8 oz.
35 B 989—State size, color.   5.98

B RAYON GABARDINE. Western made. Distinctive, embroidered two-tone style, white piping trim. Styled with snap buttons, tapered five-button cuffs. Rayon lined yoke, two piped dart-pockets, shaped body, full length tails. Dry clean. Brown with Tan, Maroon with Gray. Sizes: 14½, 15, 15½, 16-in. neck. Shipping weight 1 lb. 9 oz.
35 B 990T—State size, color.   9.98

C WOOL AND RAYON GABARDINE. wearing fabric is 23% New 77% Rayon. Rich vat-dyed colors. than 2%. Pearl snap buttons and full leng Maroon, Gray or Tan. Washabl Sizes: 14, 14½, 15, 15½, 16, 16½ neck. Shipping weight 1 lb. 9 oz.
35 B 902—State size and color.

D COTTON DENIM. Made in the West. Long-wearing. Sanforized —shrinks less than 1%. Two Arizona flap pockets and shoulder yoke, 3-snap button cuffs, full length tails. Washable. Sizes: 14, 14½, 15, 15½, 16, 16½, 17-in. neck. To Measure, below right.
35 B 981—Pearl snap buttons.   4.98
35 B 980—Enameled buttons.   3.87

E CORD-WOVEN COMBED COTTON. Vat-dyed. Sanforized—shrinks less than 1%. Two Arizona 2-point wing pockets, 3-point yoke, tapered cuffs, regular collar, pearl snap-buttons, full length tails. Washable. Colors: Blue, Green, Tan.
Half Sizes: 14, 17-in. neck. Ship. wt. 1 lb. 8 oz.
35 B 939—State size, color.   7.49

F COTTON BROADCLOTH. With Bag Pockets. Sturdy vat-d ric. Sanforized for lasting fi saddle bag pockets, tapered cuffs, full length tails, shank s Med. Blue, Med. Gray, Tan. We Sizes: 14, 14½, 15, 15½, 16, 16½, 17-i Measure, below. Wt. 1 lb. 2 oz.
35 B 952—State size, color.....

G RAYON GABARDINE. Tailored in classic Western style. Vat-dyed, pre-shrunk fabric shrinks less than 3%. Has regular collar, two one-button flap pockets, full length tails, three-button cuffs. Washable. Gray, Tan, Maroon, Dk. Green. Sizes: 14, 14½, 15, 15½, 16, 16½, 17-in. neck. Ship. wt. 1 lb. 4 oz.
35 B 926—State size, color.   4.87

H ALL NEW WOOL Worsted Gabardine or Cotton Twill. Regular collar, three-button cuffs, ocean pearl shank buttons. Wt. 1 lb. 9 oz.
35B955T—Gabardine. Tan, Med. Blue, Gray, Dk. Brown. Dry clean.
Half Sizes: 14-17-in. neck.   11.95
35B945—Cotton Twill. Tan, Blue, Gray. Washable. Half Sizes: 14½-17-in. neck. State size, color.   3.59

MEASURE from center of collar bu ter end of buttonhole. 14, 14½-in has 33-in. sleeve; 15, 15½, sleeve; 16, 16½, 17 has 34½

SHIRTS with numbers ending in "T" ed from Chicago. Order, pay from Wards nearest Mail Order

COLORS SHOWN match actual te closely as high speed printing a

426 WARDS SAE

Western style shirts made of gabardine, denim and cotton accented
with piping and embroidery in solid-color and two-toned color
combinations. This group dates from 1950.

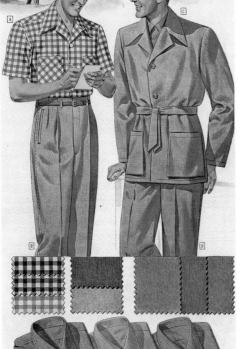

Sport denim in assorted colors dating from
the early 1950s and advertised as"...Latest in
California Casuals".

Pants

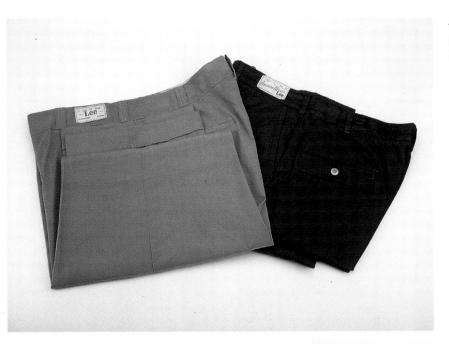

Two pair, men's, Rayon and Polyester cuffed pants labeled Leesure Wear by Lee. $45-60 pair

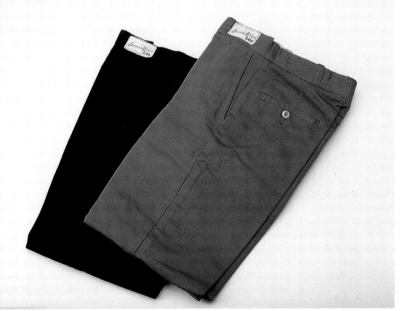

Two pair of flannel lined cotton pants with cuffs, labeled Leesure Wear by Lee. $40-50 pair

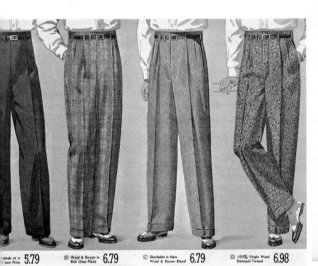

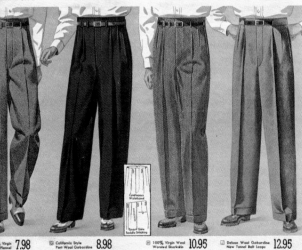

Advertised as "sporty slacks for year' round wear", these examples were offered from Spiegel in 1950.

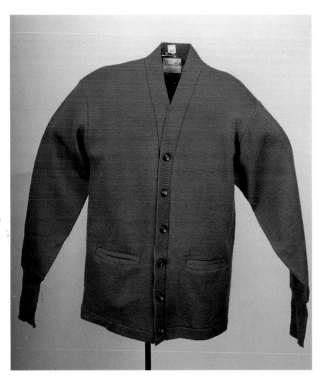

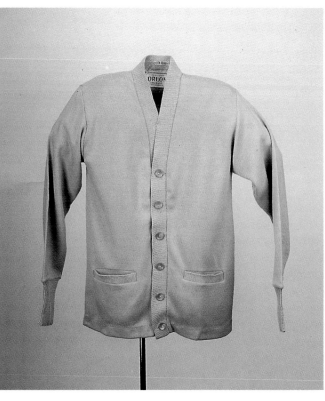

Green button down cardigan sweater made of wool, labeled Ronny-Lee Sportswear by S.Segal and Son. $30-40

Gray button down cardigan sweater made of 100% virgin orlon. No label. $30-40

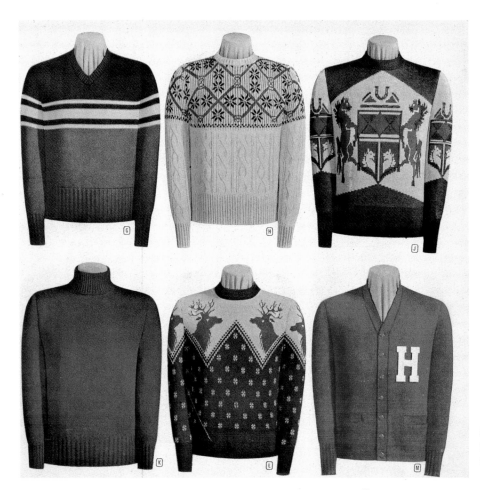

Sweaters for young men in v-neck, crew neck, turtleneck and cardigan styles from 1950.

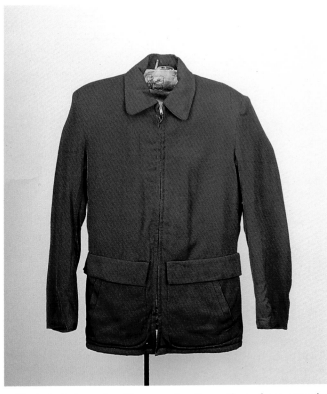

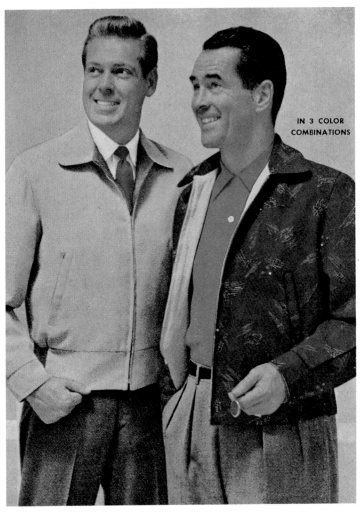

Man's jacket, made of brown gabardine with zip front, rounded collar, classic styling with cinch waist and two flap pockets, labeled A Bruce Creation. $80-125

IN 3 COLOR COMBINATIONS

Men's reversible jackets made of fortified Nylon in popular styles from 1957.

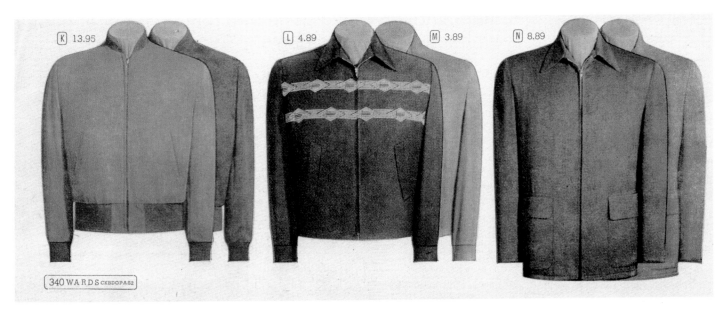

Men's sporty zip-front jackets offered for sale from Montgomery Ward in 1955.

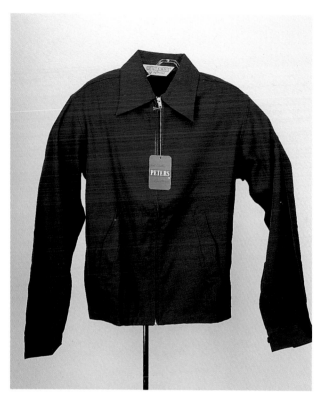

Navy blue zip front, lightweight gabardine jacket, labeled Peter's Sportswear. $50-75

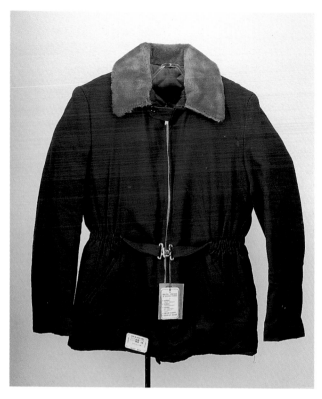

Navy blue Sur Coat made of rayon, acetate and nylon, trimmed with beaverticks, a quality pile fabric with a moth-proofed water repellent finish, manufactured by the Shelton Looms Sidney Blumenthal and Company New York. $60-85

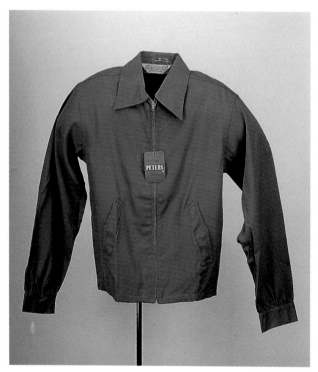

Man's jacket with zip front and pointed collar, made of rayon and acetate, labeled Peter's Sportswear Co. Philadelphia, PA. $35-50

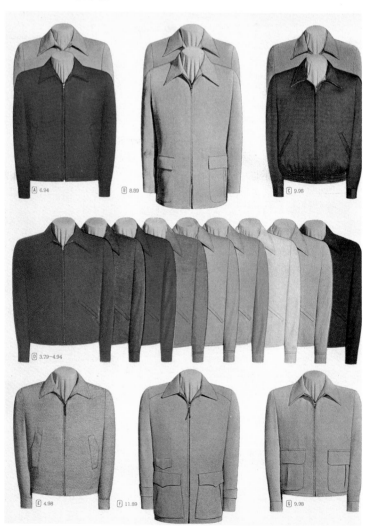

Gabardine jackets for men available in a wide range of colors and styles offered from Montgomery Ward in 1953.

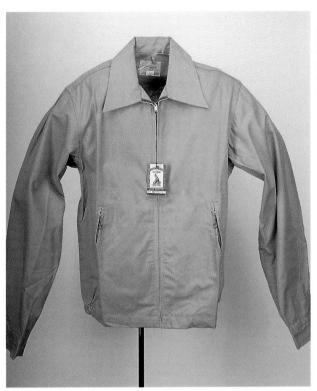

All-weather zip front jacket, labeled Town Topic. Original tag reads: Weather-sealed by Impreonole Laboratory Certified Water Repellent. $40-50

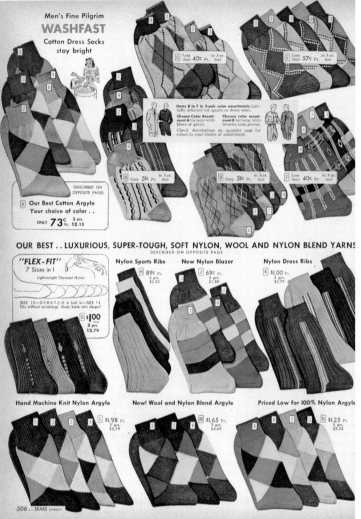

Sears brand "Pilgrim" socks for men in solids, argyles and stripes made of cotton and nylon dating from 1953.

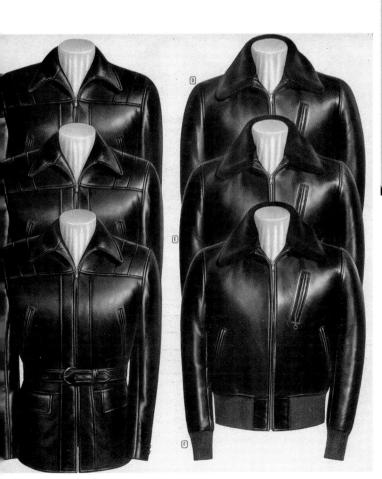

Surcoats and flight jackets from 1950 made of horsehide, cowhide and mountain cape skin.

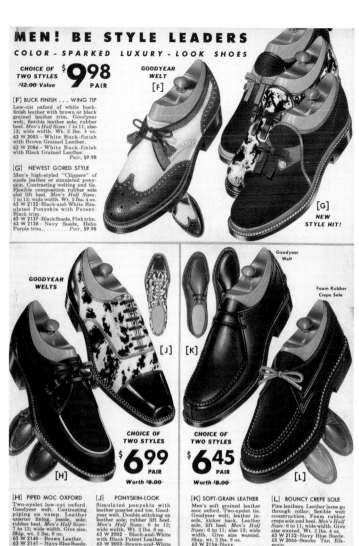

MEN! BE STYLE LEADERS
COLOR-SPARKED LUXURY-LOOK SHOES

CHOICE OF TWO STYLES **$9⁹⁸** PAIR
$12.00 Value

GOODYEAR WELT [F]

[F] BUCK FINISH . . . WING TIP
Low-cut oxford of white buck-finish leather with brown or black grained leather trim. Goodyear welt; flexible leather sole; rubber heel. *Men's Half Sizes:* 7 to 11; also 12; wide width. Wt. 2 lbs. 4 oz.
63 W 2085—White Buck-finish with Brown Grained Leather.
63 W 2086—White Buck-finish with Black Grained Leather.
Pair, $9.98

[G] NEWEST GORED STYLE
Men's high-styled "Clippers" of suede leather or simulated pony-skin. Contrasting welting and tie. Flexible composition rubber sole and lift heel. *Men's Half Sizes:* 7 to 12; wide width. Wt. 2 lbs. 4 oz.
63 W 2132—Black-and-White Simulated Ponyskin with Patent-Black trim.
63 W 2137—Black Suede, Pink trim.
63 W 2138—Navy Suede, Helio Purple trim. . . . . *Pair, $9.98*

[G] NEW STYLE HIT!

GOODYEAR WELTS [H]

[J] [K] Goodyear Welt

Foam Rubber Crepe Sole

CHOICE OF TWO STYLES **$6⁹⁹** PAIR
Worth $9.00

CHOICE OF TWO STYLES **$6⁴⁵** PAIR
Worth $8.00

[L]

[H] PIPED MOC OXFORD
Two-eyelet low-cut oxford. Goodyear welt. Contrasting piping on vamp. Leather quarter lining, insole, sole; rubber heel. *Men's Half Sizes:* 7 to 12; wide width. Give size. Ship. wt. 2 lbs. 8 oz.
63 W 2140—Brown Leather.
63 W 2141—Navy Blue Suede.
63 W 2142—Charcoal Gray Leather. . . . . *Pair, $6.99*

[J] PONYSKIN-LOOK
Simulated ponyskin with leather quarter and toe. Goodyear welt. Double stitching on leather sole; rubber lift heel. *Men's Half Sizes:* 6 to 12; wide width. Wt. 2 lbs. 8 oz.
63 W 2002—Black-and-White with Black Patent Leather.
63 W 2003—Brown-and-White with Brown smooth Leather.
Pair, $6.99

[K] SOFT-GRAIN LEATHER
Men's soft grained leather moc oxford. Two-eyelet tie. Goodyear welt; leather insole, kicker back. Leather sole, lift heel. *Men's Half Sizes:* 6 to 12; also 12; wide width. Give size wanted. Ship. wt. 2 lbs. 8 oz.
63 W 2154—Navy.
63 W 2153—Golden Tan.
63 W 2159—Black. *Pr., $6.45*

[L] BOUNCY CREPE SOLE
Fine leathers. Leather laces go through collar; flexible welt construction. Foam rubber crepe sole and heel. *Men's Half Sizes:* 6 to 11; wide width. Give size wanted. Wt. 2 lbs. 4 oz.
63 W 2152—Navy Blue Suede.
63 W 2066—Smoke Tan Elkgrain.
63 W 2067—Golden brown Elkgrain. . . . . *Pair, $6.45*

227

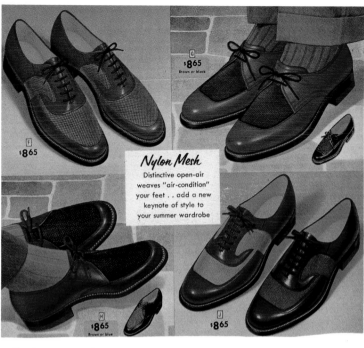

[F] $8⁶⁵
[G] Brown or black $8⁶⁵

Nylon Mesh
Distinctive open-air weaves "air-condition" your feet . . add a new keynote of style to your summer wardrobe

[H] $8⁶⁵ Brown or blue
[J] $8⁶⁵

Men's summer dress shoes made of leather and nylon mesh, popular in the 1950s.

Unusual styles in men's shoes offered for sale from the National Bellas Hess Company in the Summer of 1955. The simulated pony skin shoe was sure to be an attention-getter!

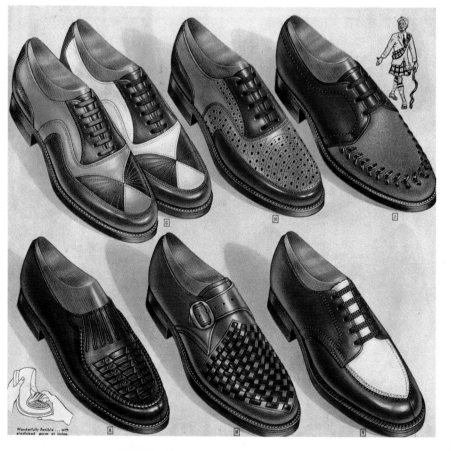

Classy assortment of men's shoes advertised as"...the newest designs by Jock McGregor" from 1950.

Chapter IV
Fashions for Boys

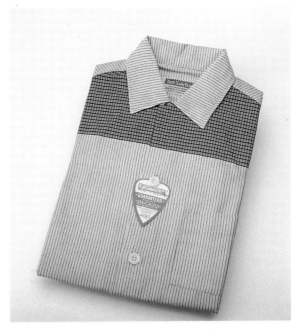

Three-toned cotton shirt with a combination of stripes and checks, and a widespread collar, labeled Tom Sawyer. $15-20 each

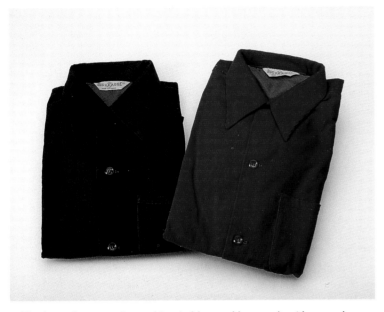

Two long sleeve corduroy shirts in blue and burgundy with spread collars, labeled Big League. $25-35 each

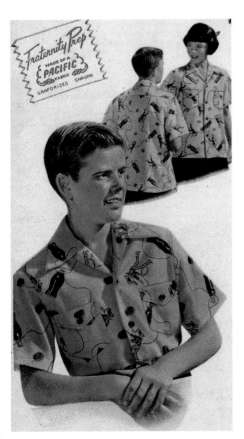

Western-style "Coca-Cola" shirt made of sanforized cotton by Fraternity Prep offered for sale from Sears. This shirt was suitable for either boys or girls.

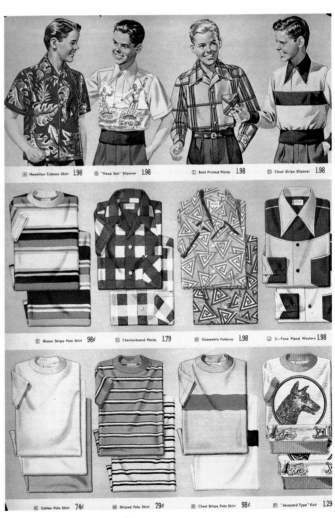

Variety of boy's shirts in button-down and pull-over styles offered for sale in 1951.

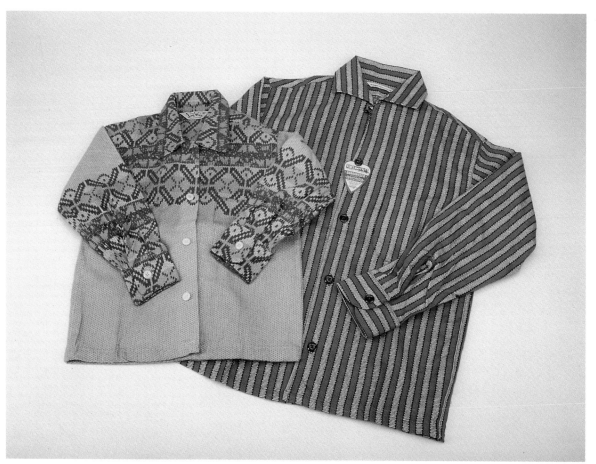

Two, boy's, cotton flannel shirts, one with a geometric border print and grey body, labeled Sparten's Jay Vees. The other with vertical stripes in a brown and grey pattern, labeled Tom Sawyer. $15-25 each

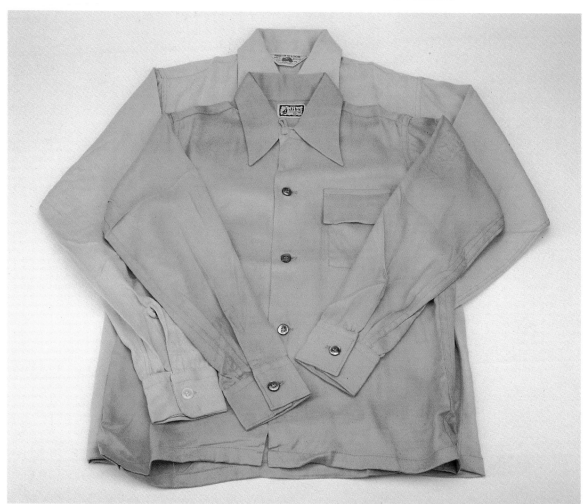

Two, boy's, long sleeve gabardine shirts with flap pockets, one labeled Jibs Juvenile, and the other labeled Fruit of the Loom Sportswear. $25-35 each

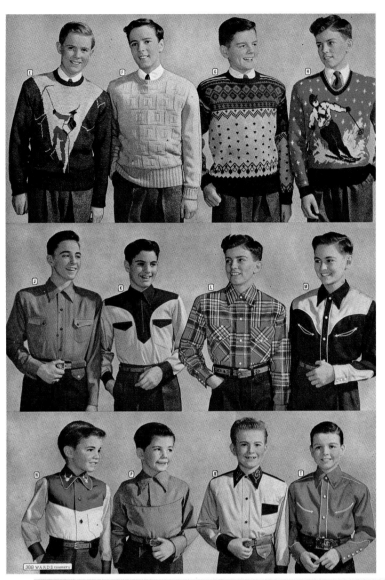

Colorful sweaters in solid colors and novelty knits in addition to western-style shirts trimmed with piping and embroidery fashionable in 1950.

Three identical cotton shirts with plaid designs in different color combinations, labeled Wrinkl-Shed, It's a Dan River Cotton. $15-20 each

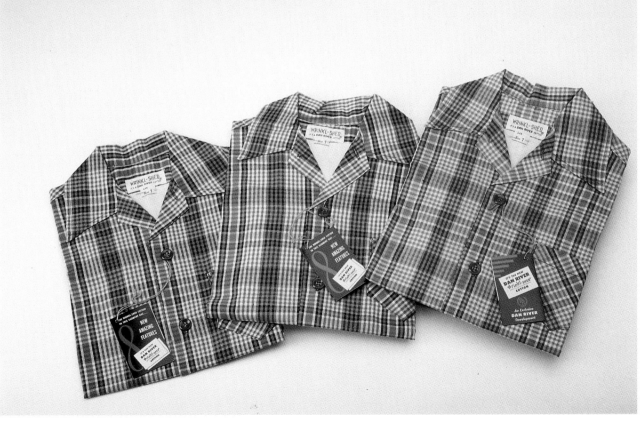

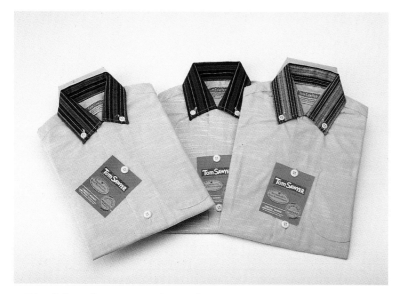

Trio of short sleeve cotton shirts with striped, button-down collars, labeled Tom Sawyer Apparel for Real Boys. $15-20 each

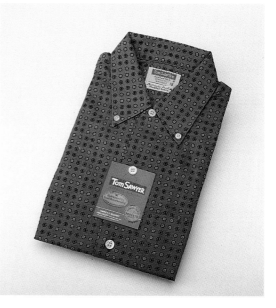

Cotton shirt with three-toned geometric print, designed with button down collar, labeled Tom Sawyer Authentic English Madder Tones. $15-20 each

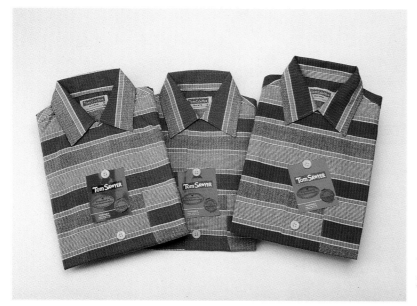

Three cotton shirts with horizontal and vertical striping in different color combinations, labeled Tom Sawyer. $18-25 each

Three shirts with small prints in different color combinations, made of cotton, designed with button down collars, labeled Kaynee Crest of Quality. $15-20 each

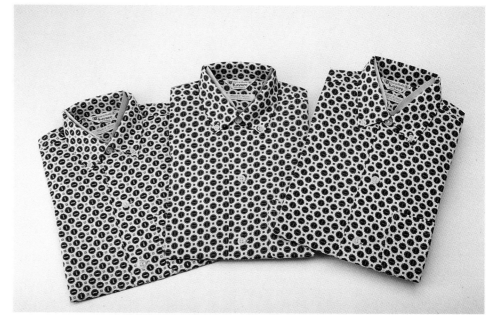

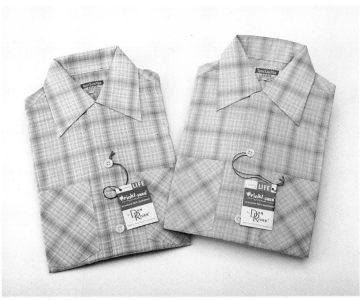

Two plaid shirts in popular 1950s color combinations, labeled Tom Sawyer. $22-28 each

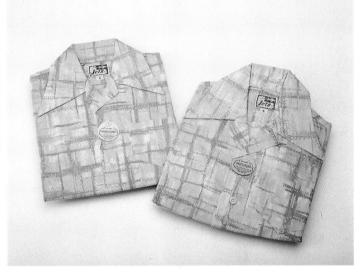

Two short-sleeved cotton shirts with splash checked prints, labeled Jets. $25-30 each

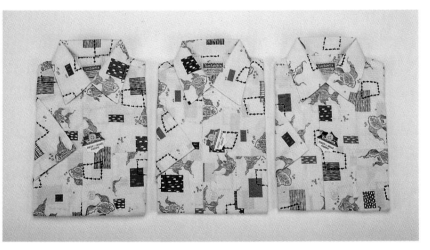

Three identical short-sleeved shirts for boys in different color combinations with a fish motif, made of cotton with a rippled texture, labeled Tom Sawyer. $25-30 each

Two identical cotton shirts in different color combinations with heraldic designs, labeled Kaynee Crest of Quality. $15-20 each

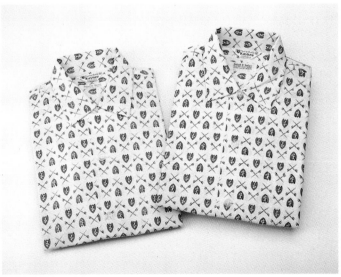

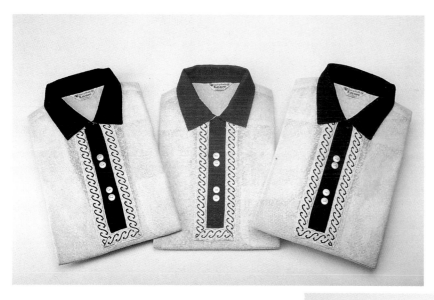

Three open-weave knit shirts with metallic thread decoration in different color combinations, labeled Kaynee Crest of Quality. $20-25 each

Four knit shirts made of wash n' wear jersey by Allen, labeled Knitted Fashions by Kaynee. $12-18 each

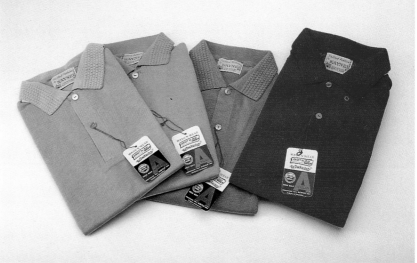

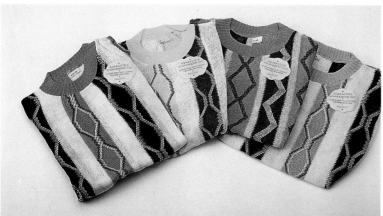

Four cable knit pullovers with zig-zag patterns, made of cotton. Tag reads: Guaranteed Genuine Raschel Knit, Made of the Finest Select Combed Yarn for Long Wear. $20-30 each

Two knit shirts for boys made of combed cotton and designed with a solid color V-neckline and contrasting collar, labeled Play Togs by Gallant. Presented with their original box. $15-20 each

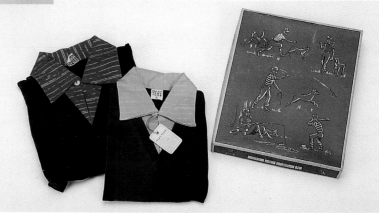

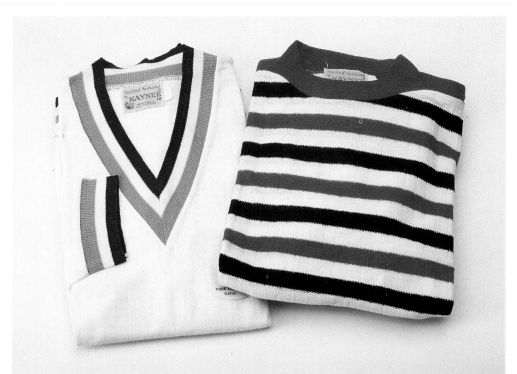

Two knitted pullovers; one with a rounded collar, the other with a V-neck, accented with three-toned stripes, labeled Kaynee. $5-10 each

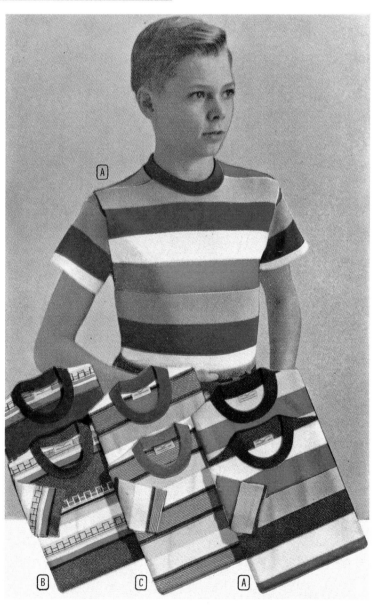

Boy's knit polo shirts in assorted striped patterns and color combinations which were popular in 1957.

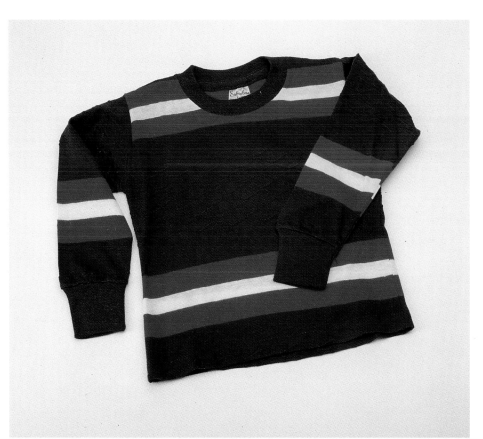

Red, white and green, long sleeve, striped polo shirt, labeled Suburban. $6-10

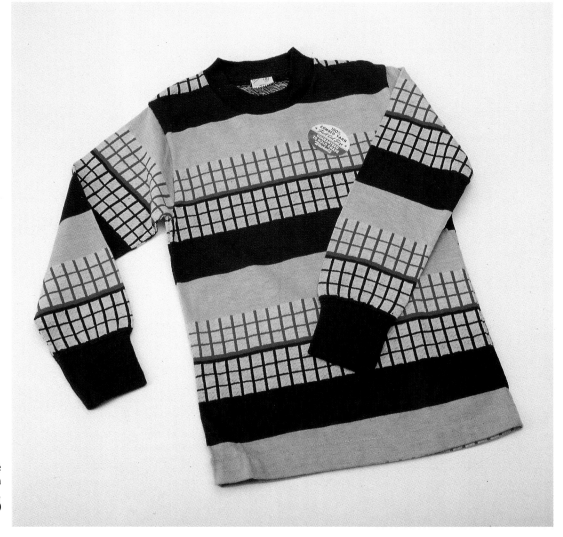

Long sleeve polo shirt made of combed cotton with striped and checked design, labeled Sterntex. $6-10

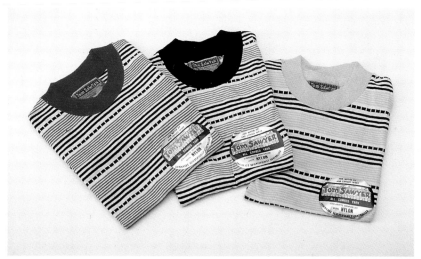

Trio of striped polo shirts, made of combed cotton. The paper label reads, "Collarette reinforced with nylon," labeled Tom Sawyer. $5-10 each

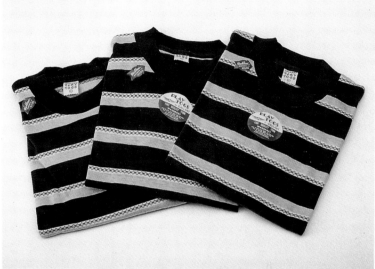

Three striped polo shirts in different color combinations, labeled Playtogs. $5-10 each

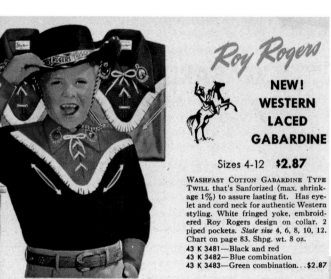

Roy Rogers

NEW! WESTERN LACED GABARDINE

Sizes 4-12 **$2.87**

WASHFAST COTTON GABARDINE TYPE TWILL that's Sanforized (max. shrinkage 1%) to assure lasting fit. Has eyelet and cord neck for authentic Western styling. White fringed yoke, embroidered Roy Rogers design on collar. 2 piped pockets. *State size* 4, 6, 8, 10, 12. Chart on page 83. Shpg. wt. 8 oz.
43 K 3481—Black and red
43 K 3482—Blue combination
43 K 3483—Green combination...$2.87

For the little buckaroo, this "Roy Rogers Western Laced Gabardine Shirt" was advertised for sale in 1951. The craze for western wear lasted the entire decade.

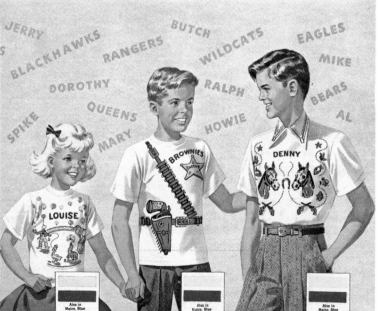

Personalized cotton knit shirts for boys and girls with circus and western themes available through mail-order catalogs in 1950.

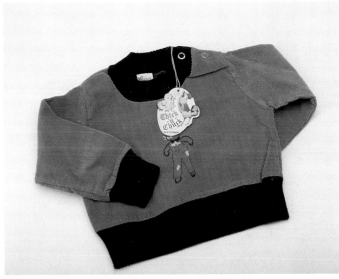

Corduroy top, "Tailored for Tots," with ribbed collar and waistband and embroidered bunny design, labeled Chick-n-Chuck. $6-10

Four corduroy tops, "Tailored for Tots," with ribbed collar and waistband and diagonal stripe, labeled Chick-n-Chuck. $8-12 each

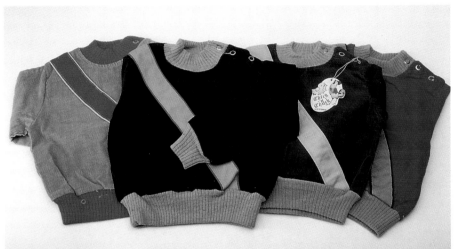

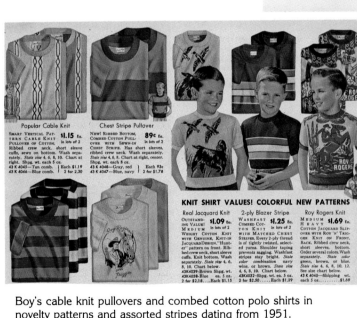

Boy's cable knit pullovers and combed cotton polo shirts in novelty patterns and assorted stripes dating from 1951.

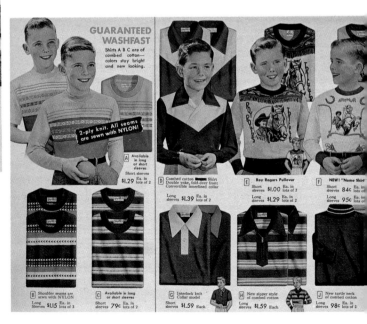

Boy's pullover shirts in stripes, solids and Western prints dating from 1953.

Sweaters

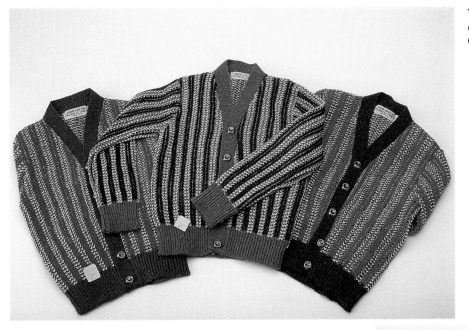

Three identical cardigan sweaters in different color combinations, labeled Made of 100% Orlon Acrylic fiber. $10-15 each

Boy's, button-down cardigan sweater with zig-zag and diamond patterns, made of 100% virgin Orlon, labeled Havenshire. $18-25

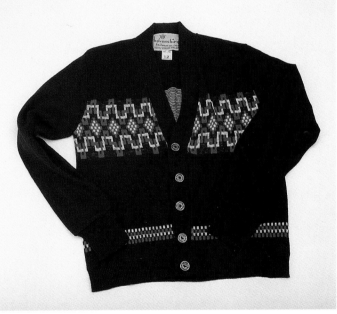

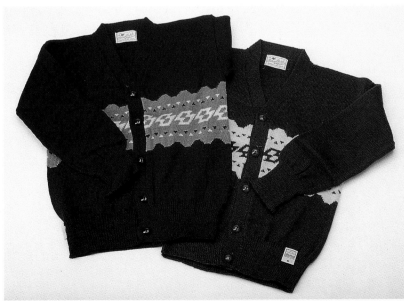

Two button down cardigan sweaters in two-toned and three-toned color combinations made of pure wool, labeled Bluebird. $18-25 each

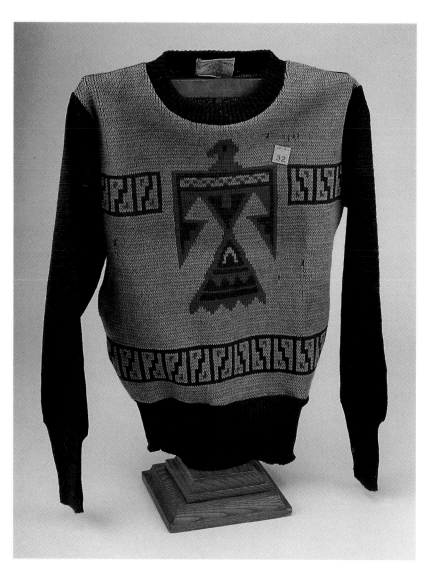

Boy's knit sweater made of wool with thunderbird design, labeled Schofield Products Sportswear. $40-50

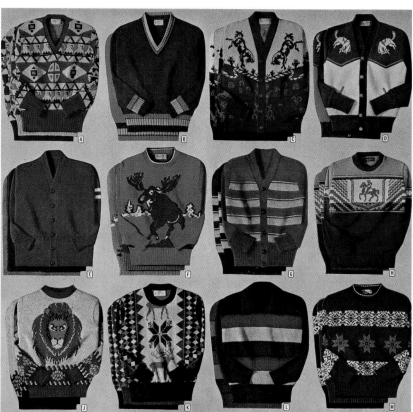

Colorful array of stylish sweaters for boys in v-neck, crew neck and cardigan styles offered for sale in 1950.

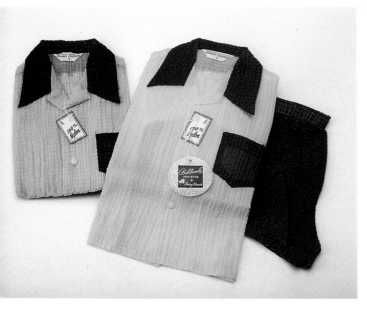

Two identical outfits in different color combinations made of textured nylon, labeled Tommy Tucker. $25-30

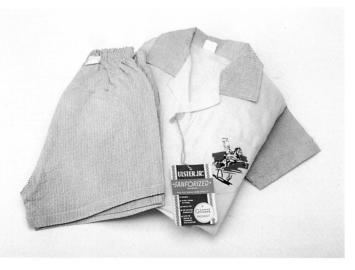

Two-piece shorts outfit made of crinkled cotton, decorated with a handpainted western motif on shirt pocket, labeled Ulster Jr. $20-30 set

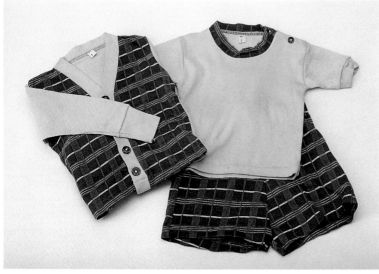

Three-piece outfit made of combed cotton consisting of shorts, pull-over shirt, and button-down cardigan. $25-30 set

Two-toned play sets, Western sets, denim shorts and polo shirts offered for sale in the summer of 1950.

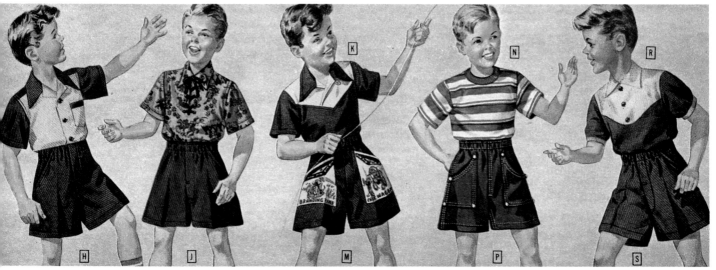

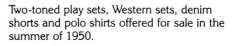

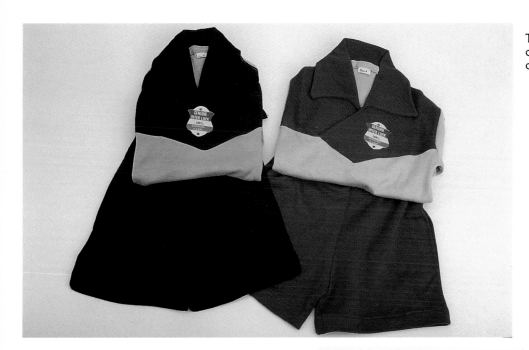

Two sets of boy's shorts and shirts of combed cotton in two-toned color combinations. $20-30 set

Two toddler boy's outfits made of combed cotton with printed shirts and solid color bottoms in different color combinations. $20-25 set

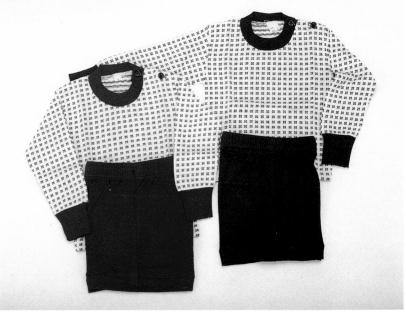

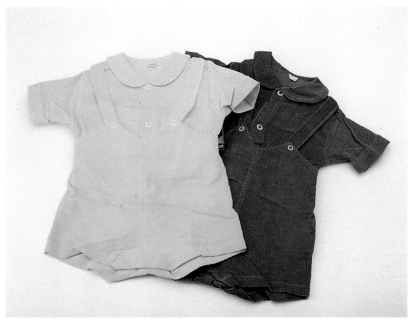

Identical two-piece cotton corduroy outfits for toddlers, in blue and yellow cotton, no labels. $18-25 set

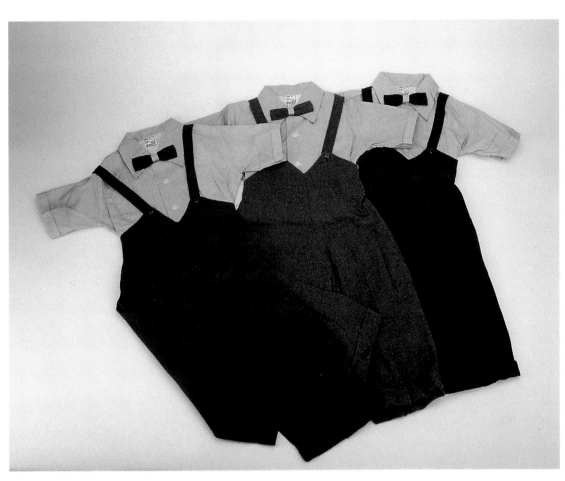

Three, little boy's dressy outfits consisting of woolen suspender pants, cotton shirts, and matching bow ties, labeled Gay Lad Togs. $25-35 set

Two, three-piece shorts outfits made of cotton and wool, with matching bow ties, labeled Master Jim. $25-30 set

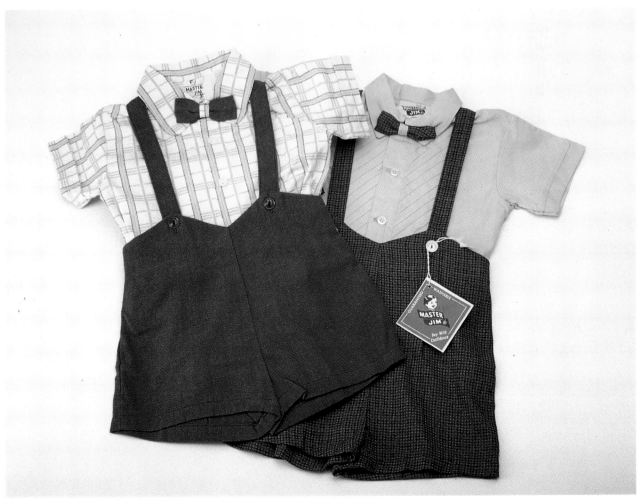

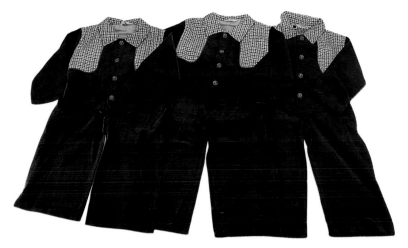

Three, cotton corduroy suits for little boys, available in different color combinations of the same design, labeled Tom Thumb. $30-40 set

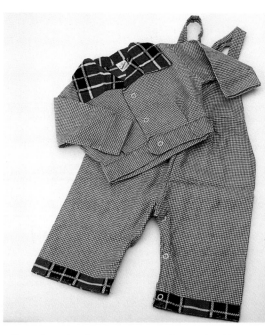

Two-piece, boy's cotton suspender outfit with plaid flannel lining, labeled KamTee. $30-40

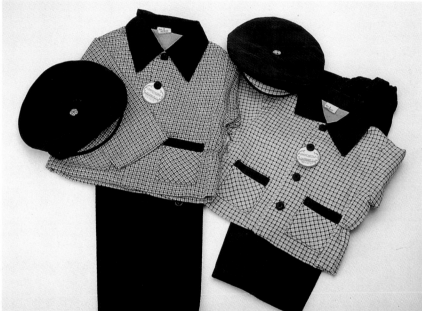

Boy's three-piece dress suits consisting of jacket, pants and matching cap in blue and green color combinations, no label. $40-50 set

Boy's assorted denims, bib overalls, coveralls and Western styled slack sets offered for sale in the 1949-1950 Fall and Winter Montgomery Ward catalog.

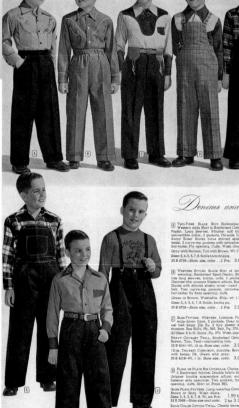

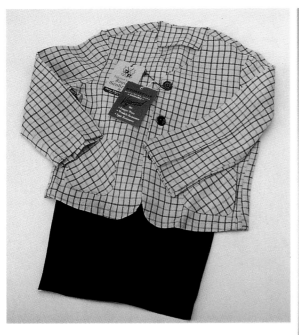

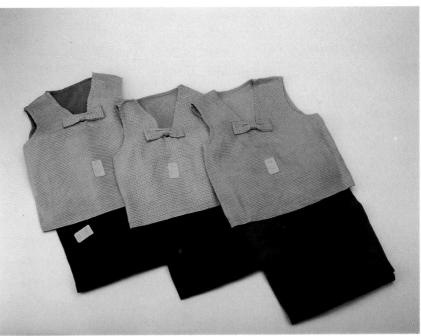

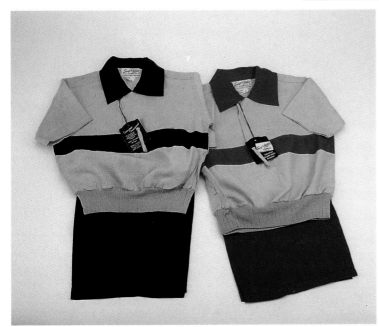

Top left: Summer dress outfit made with green Rayon gabardine suspender shorts and three-toned plaid collarless jacket, labeled Tailored for the Junior Gentleman by Philip Schneider & Co., New York. $25-35

Top right: Dress outfits for little boys, designed with solid color gabardine pants and houndstooth vests with attached bow-tie, no labels. $25-35 set

Two, boy's, cotton summer shorts and shirts sets labeled Soap 'n' Water fabric, Washable. $20-30 set

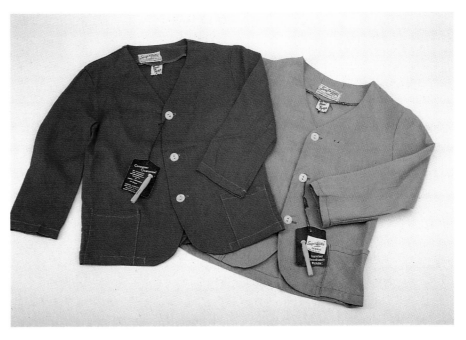

Two, boy's, summer cotton jackets labeled Soap 'n' Water fabric Washable and Toni Togs. $15-20 each

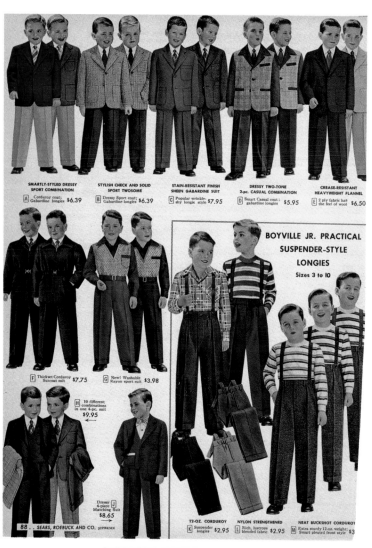

Little boy's dress suits, sport suits and suspender-style "longies" made of flannel, gabardine and corduroy available from Sears in 1953.

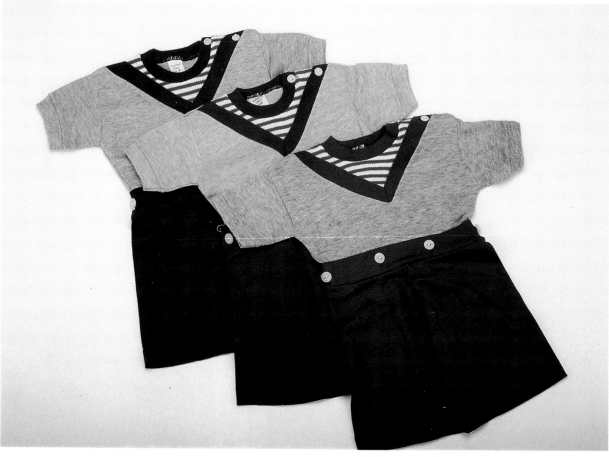

Three identical boy's two-piece outfits made of combed cotton utilizing different color combinations. The shirts are attached to the shorts with six buttons. $20-25 each set

Two toddler outfits for boys designed with cotton shirts, corduroy shorts and plaid belts, labeled My Lamb. $20-25 each

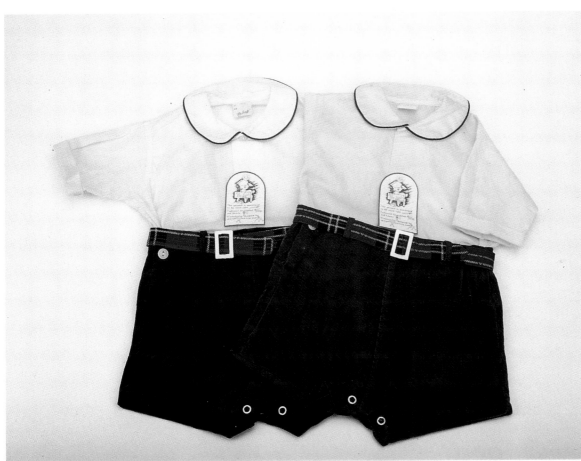

Knitted one-piece romper with matching hat made of cotton and rayon with embroidered accents, labeled Sterling Children's Wear. $20-25 set

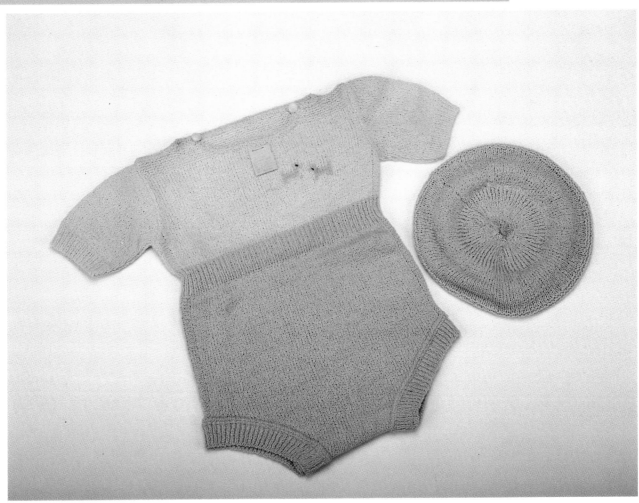

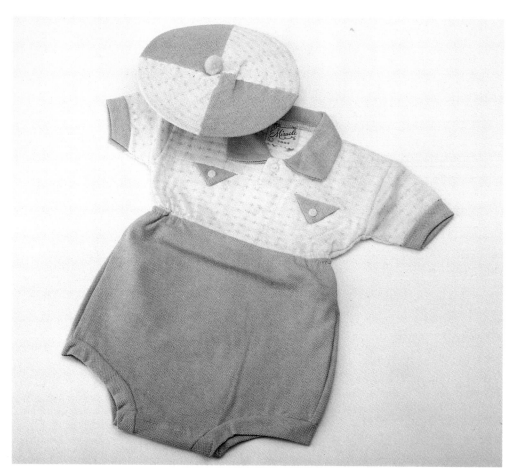

Two-toned cotton romper with matching hat, labeled Miracle Togs. $18-25 set

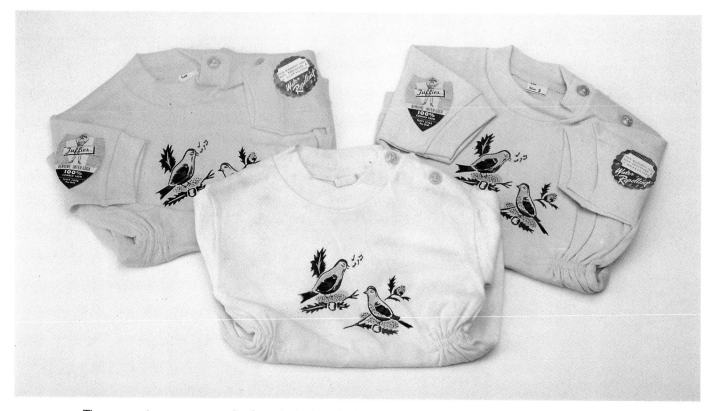

Three, one-piece rompers made of inter-locked combed cotton decorated with hand painted bird designs, labeled Tubby Togs, New York. $12-18 each

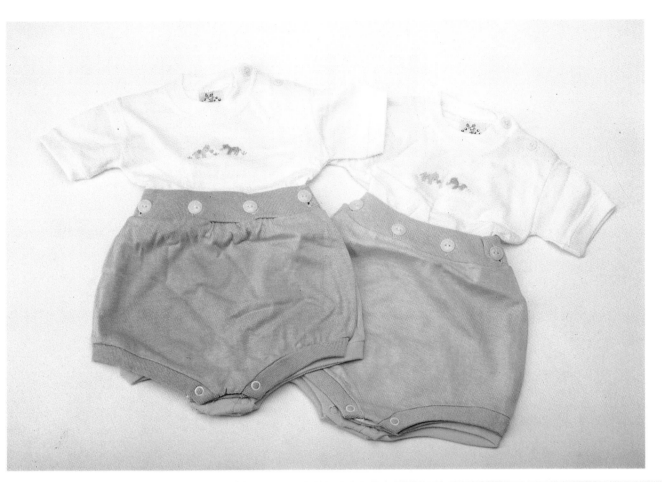

Two toddler's romper sets designed with interchangeable bottoms made of combed cotton accented with embroidered decoration. $12-18 each

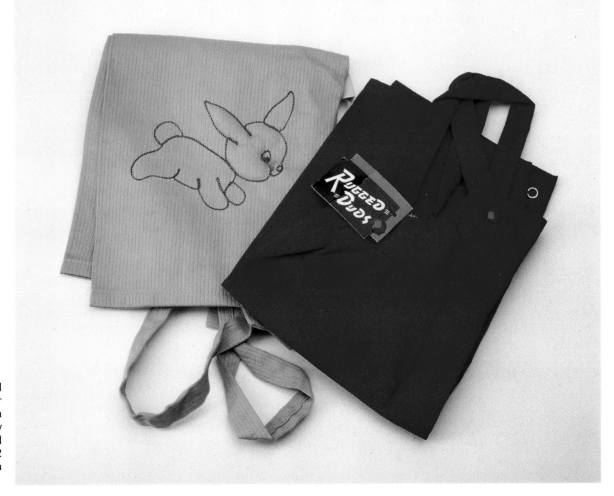

Two pair of ribbed cotton bib overalls for toddlers with embroidered bunny design, labeled Rugged Duds. $8-12 each

Pants

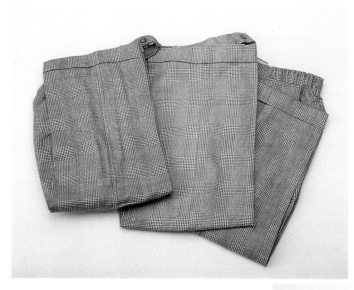

Three pair of pants with checked design and cuffed bottoms, no label $15-20 each pair

Three pair of striped denim pants with zippered fronts and buckled backs, labeled Leesure Wear by Lee. $35-45 pair

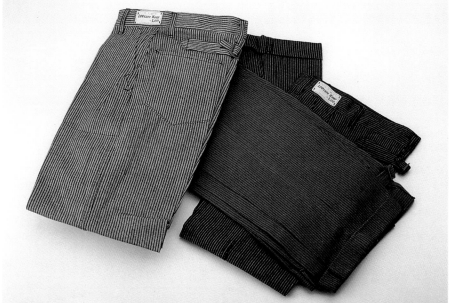

Bottom left: "Longies" for junior boys made of cotton, corduroy and nylon blend gabardines in solid colors, checks and plaids popular in 1953.

Bottom right: Slack suits and short sets made of combed cotton, gabardine, cotton plisse and seersucker popular in 1953.

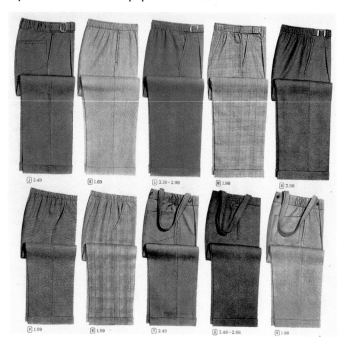

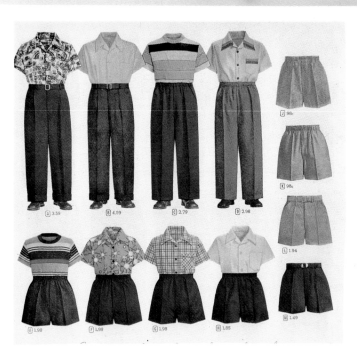

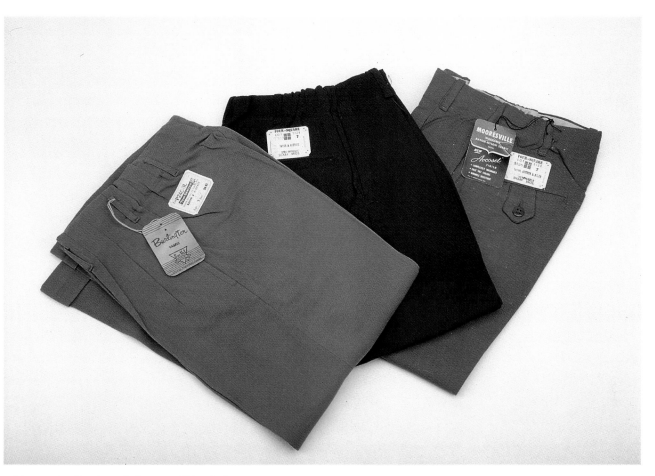

Three pair of boy's cuffed pants of blended
Rayon, Acetate, and Nylon fabric, labeled
Four-Square and Sharp Bros. $25-30 pair

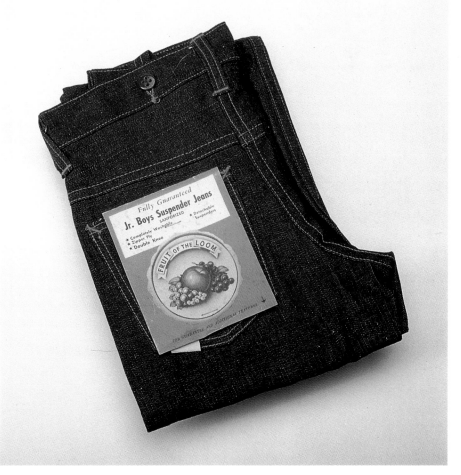

Boys' suspender jeans guaranteed
completely washable, and designed with a
zipper fly, detachable suspenders, labeled
Fruit of the Loom. $50-75

Two pair of boys'
dungarees, labeled C. C.
Brand. $30-50 each

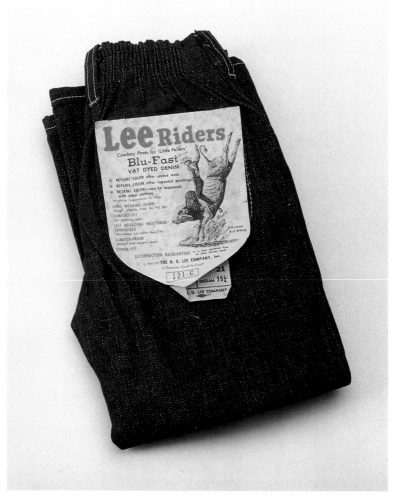

Cowboy pants for "Little Fellers"
made of vat dyed denim, labeled
H. D. Lee Co. $75-100

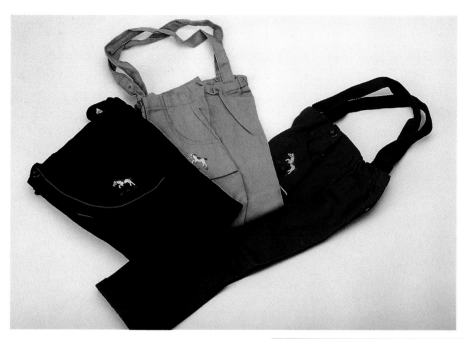

Three pair of jodhpurs of different color combinations with Western designs embroidered on the pockets. $35-45 each

Boy's jodhpurs with button-on suspenders, red piping, and side leg zippers, labeled Windsor Togs. $30-40

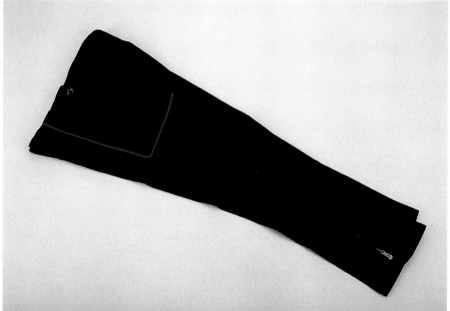

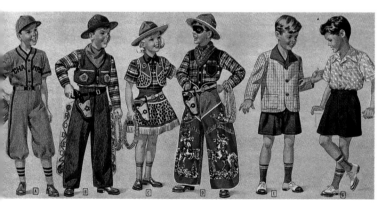

Novelty and dress outfits for children popular in 1950.

Western boots and rugged outdoor styles designed for boys made of fine grained leather advertised for sale in 1953.

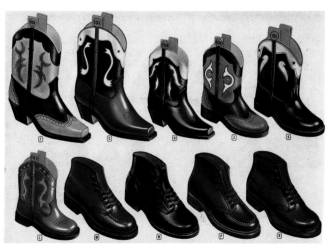

143

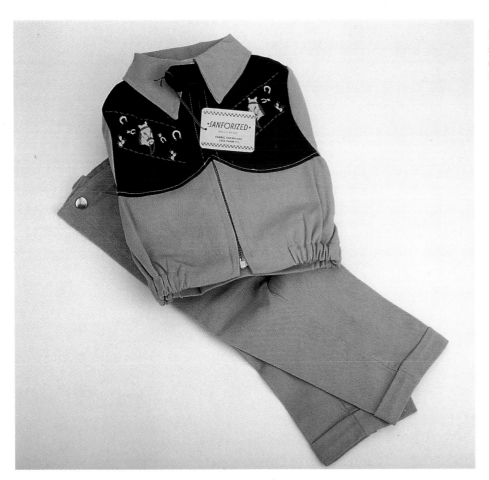

Boy's, Sanforized cotton, two-piece Western style play suit with embroidered cowboy decoration, labeled Playland Sportswear. $75-100 set

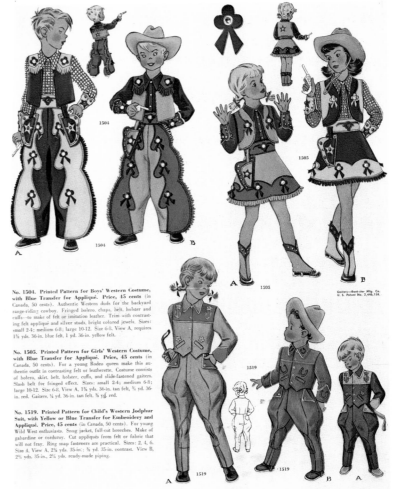

Period advertisement to purchase McCall's printed patterns for making authentic novelty Western costumes for children. Patterns for everything from chaps to jodhpurs to slide-fastened gaiters were offered to construct complete costumes for "Wild West" enthusiasts.

No. 1504. Printed Pattern for Boys' Western Costume, with Blue Transfer for Appliqué. Price, 45 cents (in Canada, 50 cents). Authentic Western duds for the backyard range-riding cowboy. Fringed bolero, chaps, belt, holster and cuffs—to make of felt or imitation leather. Trim with contrasting felt appliqué and silver studs, bright colored jewels. Sizes: small 2-4; medium 6-8; large 10-12. Size 6-8, View A, requires 1⅝ yds. 36-in. blue felt, 1 yd. 36-in. yellow felt.

No. 1505. Printed Pattern for Girls' Western Costume, with Blue Transfer for Appliqué. Price, 45 cents (in Canada, 50 cents). For a young Rodeo queen make this authentic outfit in contrasting felt or leatherette. Costume consists of bolero, skirt, belt, holster, cuffs, and slide-fastened gaiters. Slash belt for fringed effect. Sizes: small 2-4; medium 6-8; large 10-12. Size 6-8, View A, 1⅞ yds. 36-in. tan felt, ¾ yd. 36-in. red. Gaiters, ¼ yd. 36-in. tan felt, ⅜ yd. red.

No. 1519. Printed Pattern for Child's Western Jodhpur Suit, with Yellow or Blue Transfer for Embroidery and Appliqué. Price, 45 cents (in Canada, 50 cents). For young Wild West enthusiasts. Snug jacket, full-cut breeches. Make of gabardine or corduroy. Cut appliqués from felt or fabric that will not fray. Ring snap fasteners are practical. Sizes: 2, 4, 6. Size 4, View A, 2⅜ yds. 35-in.; ⅝ yd. 35-in. contrast. View B, 2½ yds. 35-in., 2¼ yds. ready-made piping.

Night Clothes

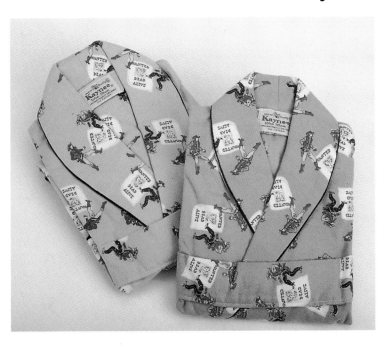

Two, boy's, cotton flannel robes with printed cowboy design, labeled Kaynee Wee Men. $35-50 each

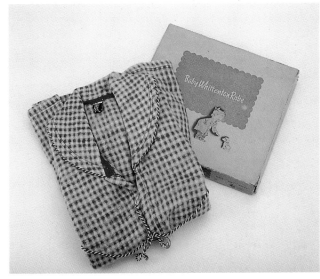

Cotton printed baby's robe by Whittenton. $25-35

Boy's, cotton flannel bathrobe with Western print and waist sash, labeled Kaynee Wee Men. $35-50

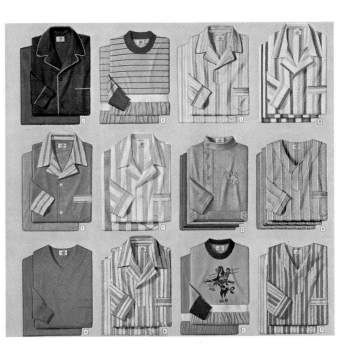

Boy's pajamas in assorted styles and fabrics featured in Wards in 1950.

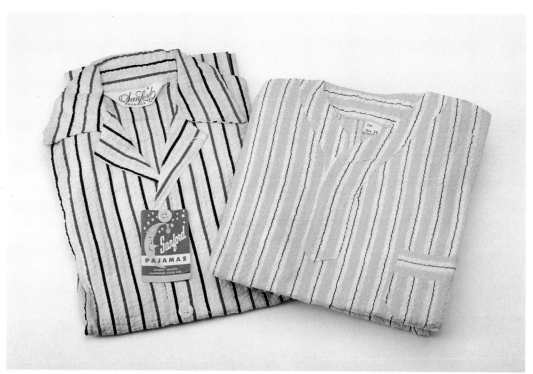

Two pair of pajamas made of crinkled cotton, with striped designs, labeled Sanford. $10-15 each

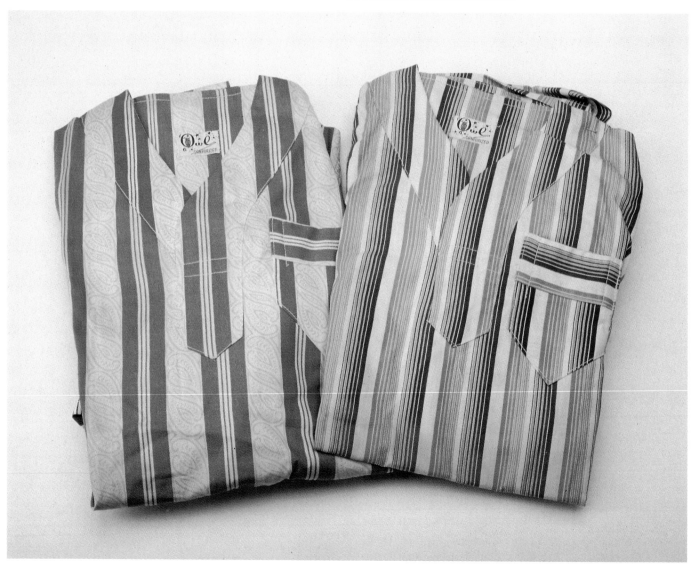

Two pair of Sanforized cotton pajamas wilth vertical striping labeled Owl. $10-15 each pair

146

Underwear

Assortment of cotton boxers with abstract and geometric prints, labeled Fruit of the Loom. $3-5 each

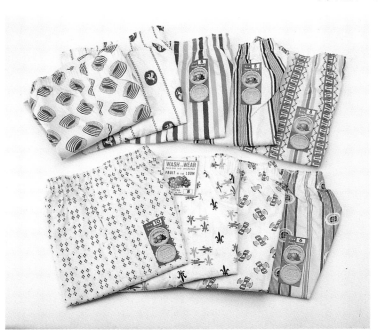

Group of men's, Sanforized cotton, printed boxer shorts by Fruit of the Loom, accompanied by their original box. $3-5 each

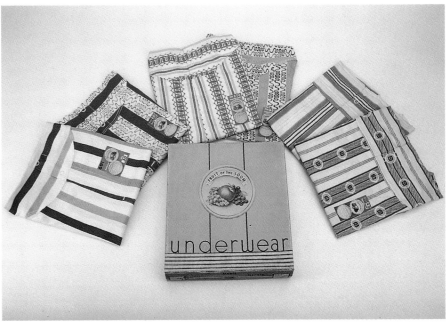

Socks

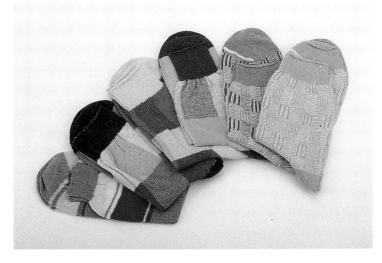

Six pair of boy's cotton socks in an assortment of colors and patterns. $2-4 each pair

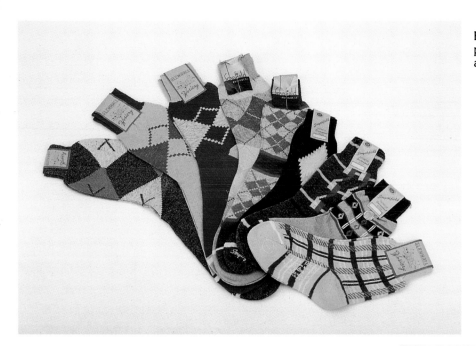

Boy's cotton socks with argyle and plaid patterns, labeled Smithfield, Glenhall, and Schofield. $2-4 each pair

Boy's cotton socks with plaid, argyle, and striped patterns. $2-4 each pair

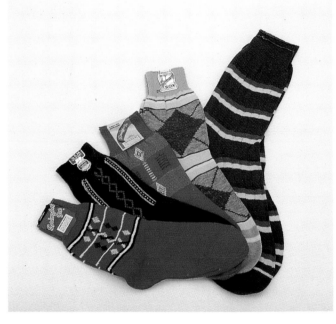

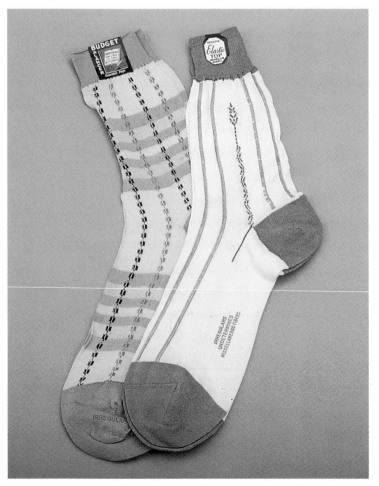

Two pair of nylon, socks; both marked "irregulars". One labeled "Undetermined Miscellaneous Fibers." $3-5 each pair

Bathing Trunks

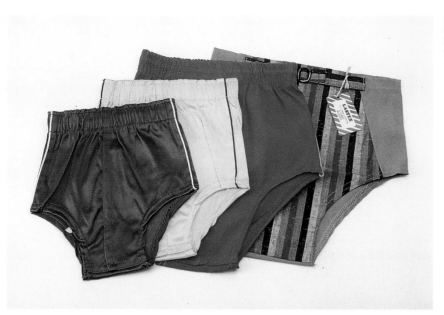

Four pair of boy's bathing trunks made of Formfit Lastex cotton and rubber. $5-10 each

Identical swim trunks in different color combinations with nautical prints, labeled Blue Bird Swimwear. $7-10 each

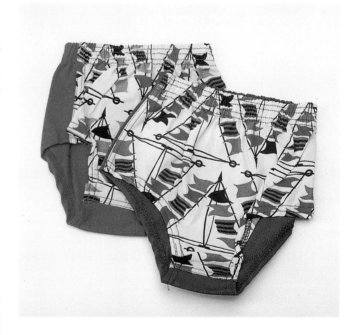

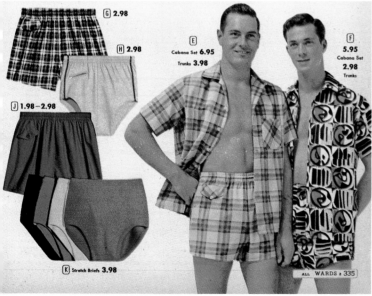

Cabana sets, swim trunks and briefs made of cotton and stretch nylon in solids and prints advertised for sale in 1957.

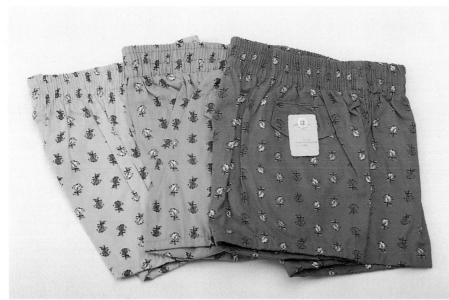

Trio of trunks designed for swim and play, made of printed cotton, labeled Kaynee. $8-12 each

Two pair of cotton swim trunks with Persian print, labeled Kaynee. $8-12 each

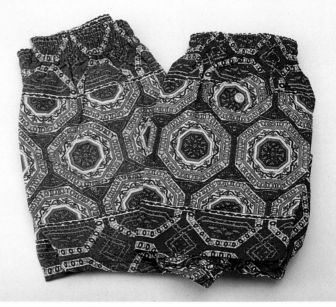

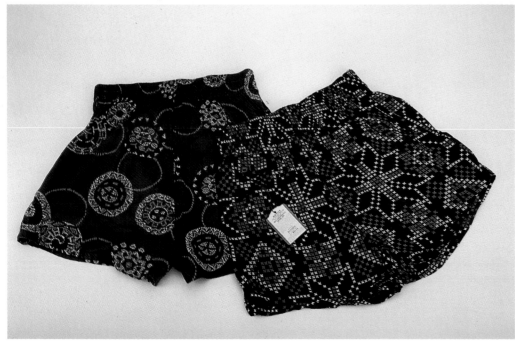

Two pair of men's swim trunks of printed Acetate and Rayon fibers, with dark blue and dark green backgrounds. $10-15 each

Shoes

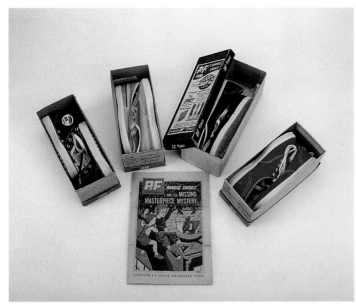

Four pair of children's P.F. Flyers canvas shoes (sneakers) with an original Adventure Book #3. $20-30 pair

Boy's original high-top P. F. Flyers by B. F. Goodrich in original box. $35-50

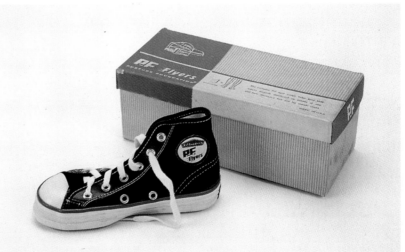

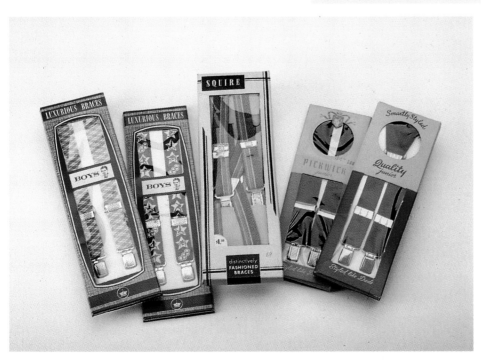

Assortment of boy's suspenders, popularly called "braces," labeled Squire and Pickwick. $8—12 each

Outer Wear

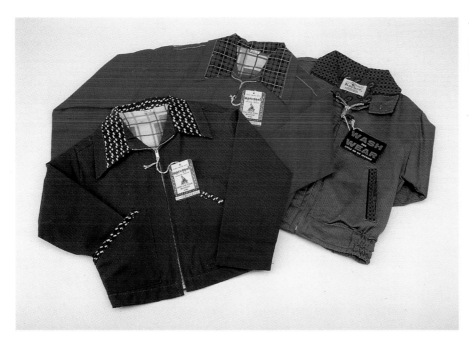

Three, boy's, cotton jackets with patterned collars and zipper front closures, labeled Impregnole and Kaynee. $30-40 each

Three, boy's, cotton jackets with zipper front closings. The red plaid bears no label, the solid red is labeled Leesure Wear by Lee, and the solid green is labeled Peter's Sportswear and Dan River Fabrics. $25-35 each

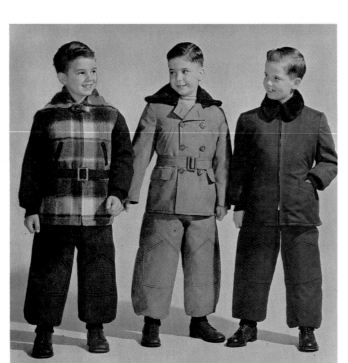

Little boy's cold-weather suits made of wool with attached hood or poplin with mouton collars stylish in the Winter of 1950-1951.

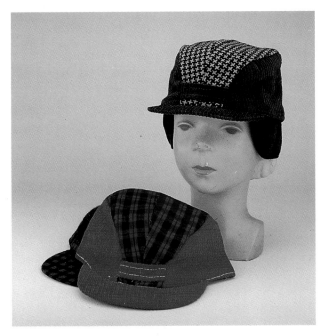

Three, boy's, cotton corduroy, winter caps with felt and quilted linings and folding ear flaps, not labeled. $8-12 each

Four, boy's, cotton corduroy, winter caps with folding ear flaps, labeled Cinderella. $8-12 each

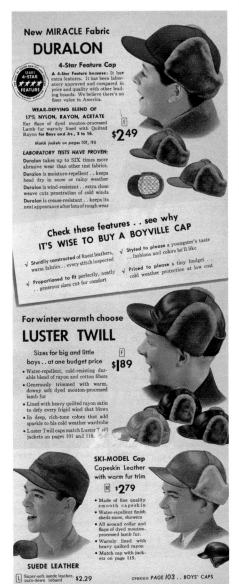

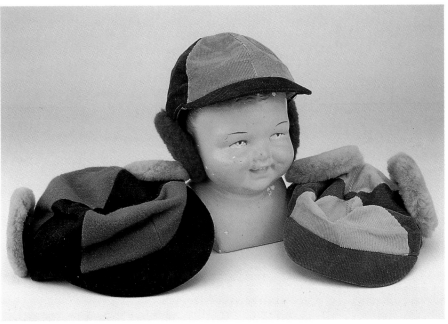

Three, boy's, winter caps with rotating ear muffs, no labels. $12-20 each

Boy's caps from 1953 made of Cape skin leather, suede, Luster Twill and Duralon.

153

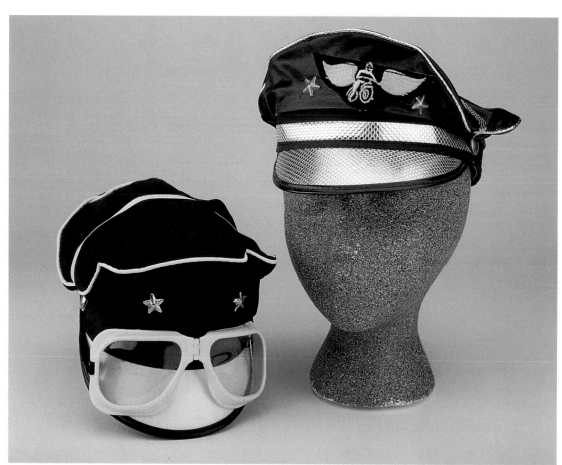

Two, boy's, motorcycle-style caps, one with attached goggles, no labels. $15-20 each

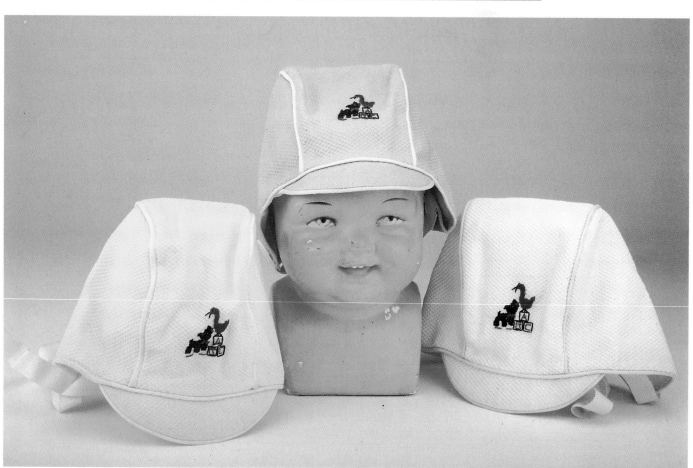

Three, baby's, cotton, summer caps with embroidered decoration, no labels. $6-10 each

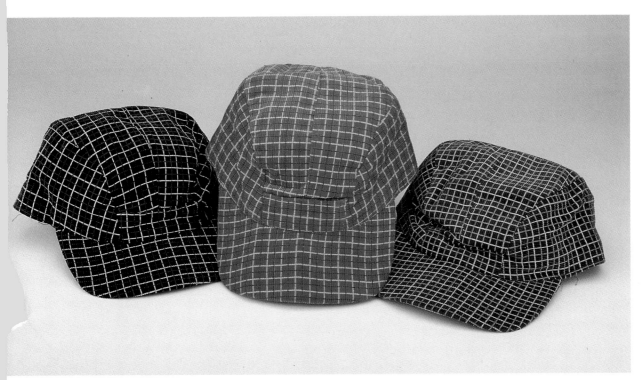

Three, boy's, cotton corduroy, plaid printed winter caps with quilted linings, no labels. $8-12 each

Four, boy's, winter caps with folding ear muffs, two in leather and two in fabric, no labels. $15-20 each

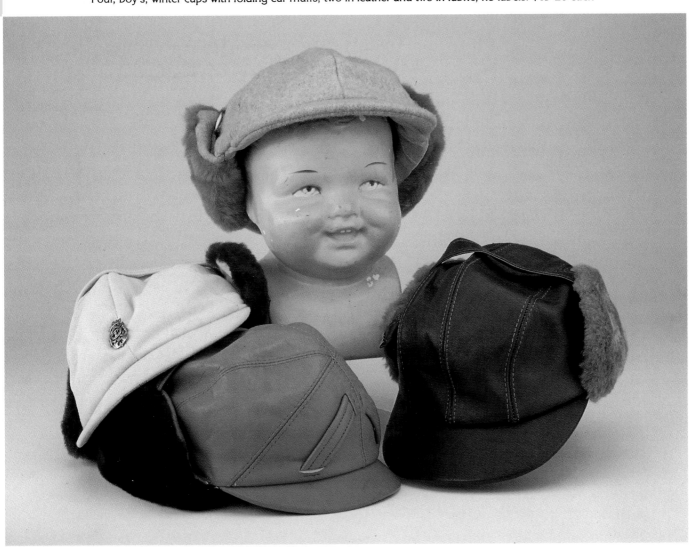

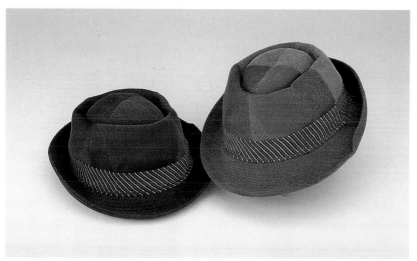

Two, boy's, corduroy dress hats with brims and folding ear flaps, no labels. $15-20 each

Two, boy's, knit and fabric caps with folding ear flaps. $15-20 each

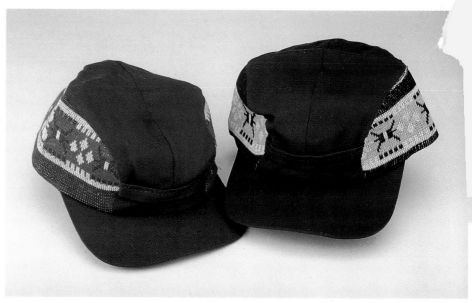

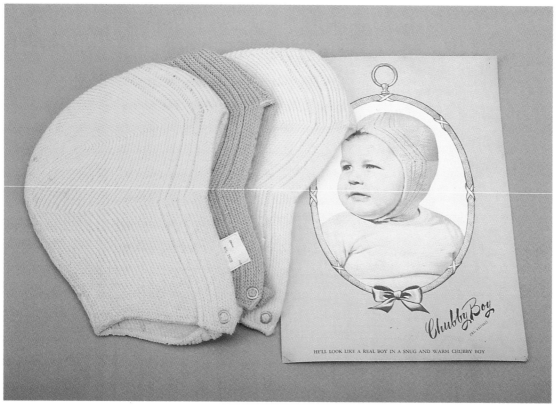

Three, wool knit, baby boy's caps in yellow, blue and white solid colors, by Chubby Boy. $8-12 each

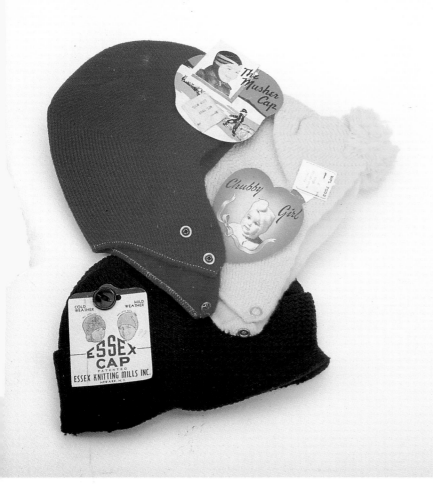

Yellow, wool, baby girl's cap by Chubby Girl. Dark blue, cotton knit, boy's cap by Essex Knitting Mills, Newark, New Jersey. Red, wool, boy's cap, labeled The Musher Cap. $8-12 each

Two muffler and glove sets made of wool with argyle and checked designs, labeled Piccadilly. $10-15 set

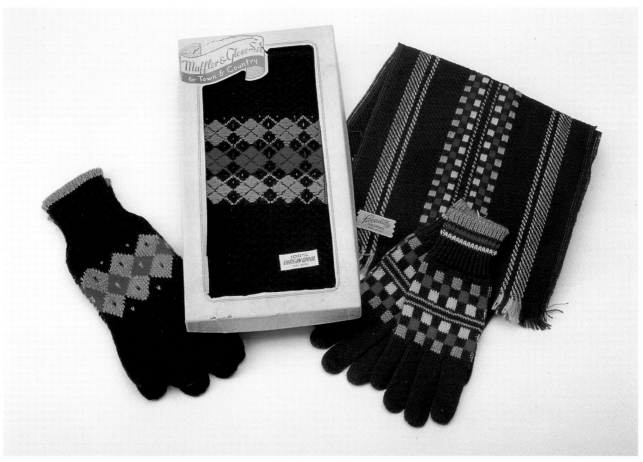

Bibliography

Catalogs

Aldens, Chicago, Illinois, Spring & Summer 1959.

Montgomery Ward, Chicago, Illinois, Fall & Winter 1949-1950, Spring & Summer 1953, Spring & Summer 1955, Spring & Summer 1957.

National Bellas Hess, Spring & Summer 1955.

Sears, Roebuck & Company, Philadelphia and Chicago, Spring & Summer 1951, Fall & Winter 1953, Spring & Summer 1955, Fall & Winter 1958.

Spiegel, Chicago, Illinois, Spring & Summer 1950, Spring & Summer 1951.

Magazines

Apparel Arts, 1955, 1956, 1957.

Charm, 1954, 1955, 1956, 1957.

Esquire, 1951, 1952, 1953, 1954, 1959.

Glamour, 1954, 1955.

Good Housekeeping, December, 1956

.Mademoiselle, 1954 and February, 1955.

Seventeen, November, 1958.